Lee ... May...

Hopefully we're all ...

This stuf

THE
OVERPARENTING
EPIDEMIC

THE
OVERPARENTING
EPIDEMIC

Why Helicopter Parenting Is Bad for Your Kids ... and Dangerous for You, Too!

George S. Glass, MD, and David Tabatsky

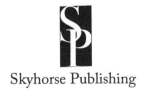

Skyhorse Publishing

Skyhorse Publishing books may be purchased in bulk at special discounts for sales promotion, corporate gifts, fund-raising, or educational purposes. Special editions can also be created to specifications. For details, contact the Special Sales Department, Skyhorse Publishing, 307 West 36th Street, 11th Floor, New York, NY 10018 or info@skyhorsepublishing.com.

Skyhorse® and Skyhorse Publishing® are registered trademarks of Skyhorse Publishing, Inc.®, a Delaware corporation.

Visit our website at www.skyhorsepublishing.com.

10 9 8 7 6 5 4 3 2 1

Library of Congress Cataloging-in-Publication Data is available on file.

Cover design by Brian Peterson

Print ISBN: 978-1-62873-730-1
Ebook ISBN: 978-1-62914-082-7

Printed in the United States of America

CONTENTS

A "QUICK-START" GUIDE

For parents living in a perpetual time crunch (aren't we all?) or simply saddled by a severe lack of concentration (perhaps caused by overparenting), we suggest an abbreviated version of this book. If your time and patience are limited, here is what we recommend, in this order:

Page xi: Our disclaimer. All levity aside, no single book can consider every child's special needs or the exact circumstances of any individual family.

Page xiii: The glossary. Skim through this, and if you recognize yourself—and admit it—it may behoove you to abandon this page altogether and read the entire book.

Page xxi: From the introduction: "If we never give our children permission to get things wrong, they're unlikely to ever learn how to get things right." Is this starting to make any sense?

Page 3: "Overparenting occurs when someone tries too hard to manage the outcome of his or her child's life, imposing his or her own expectations, often inappropriately, regardless of the child's wishes and abilities."

Page 4: "How Do You Know whether You Are Overparenting?" If you answer "yes" to some of the descriptions, find a comfortable chair and take notes. You obviously have a lot to learn.

Page 56: "Mindful Parenting"—This is key to everything.

Page 65: "Managing Expectations"—Oh, boy, don't we all need help with that?

Page 78: "Parental Aptitude Test"—Same as above. Keep that comfortable chair handy.

Page 129: "How Overparenting Affects Your Child"—This should make any parent curious.

Page 176: "How Overparenting Affects You as a Parent"—After all, it's all about you, isn't it? You're thinking about that . . . pretty sure you are. Gotcha! It's not *about* you. It's *because* of you. This book exists *because* of you! Ready or not, please proceed.

DISCLAIMER

We understand that parents of special-needs children must often pay special attention to an assortment of needs and conditions, and that some of our comments and prescriptive ideas may not be relevant to their situation. We must also recognize that for most of us, our own child (or children) may be considered to be "special-needs"; because we understand our children's individual needs and unique situation more than anyone else, we think that they should get "special" if not extra attention or care from the powers that be, at school or through the lens of a doctor.

For example, some parents want their child to be labeled as having attention-deficit/hyperactivity disorder (ADHD) so that they can get extra time on tests. Others would like to explain their child's shyness as a product of Asperger's syndrome so that they don't have to push the child to go out and become involved with his or her peers. Before anointing or accepting a "special-needs" label or diagnosis, your child should be evaluated by an expert in that field to truly determine what is going on and what the best course of action may be.

Note

The name, occupation, and geographic location of some of the individuals depicted in this book are composite portraits reflecting real people, whose specific identities have been protected. These anecdotal quotes have been culled from interviews and/or personal correspon-dence conducted by the authors, from personal peer groups, profes-sional associations, and confidential doctor-patient communications. Pseudonyms have been given and in some cases the quotes may be composites of the words of a variety of interview subjects. A com-plete list of those who have been interviewed and/or personally cor-responded with appears in the Acknowledgements.

GLOSSARY

Note: This list is alphabetical, so as not to reveal any personal history of the authors, both of whom are parents.

Blackhawk moms
Helicopter parents in attack mode, who will do anything to ensure their child's success, *regardless of the consequences* for anyone else. (First cousin to "cheerleader moms.")

Crispy kids or toasties
Children burned out by the time they get to college.

Curling parents (used in Scandinavia and some other parts of Europe)
Parents who sweep obstacles out of the way for their children.

Helicopter parents
Moms and dads who just can't stop hovering over their kids—at any age.

Hyper parents
Parents who are prone to overscheduling their kids.

Lawnmower parents (a.k.a. "snowplow parents")
Parents who attempt to remake terrain so that it works better for *their* child.

Parent bouncers

University-hired students trained to redirect adults who try to attend their children's classes and activities.

Satellite parents

Helicopter parents only from a distance, such as on cell phones and with video monitors.

Smothering mothering

Does this really need to be explained?

Soccer mom

An overly involved parent who tends to forget her own life.

Stealth parents

Parents who are there, still intervening, even though you can't see them.

Submarine parents

Moms and dads who undermine their children.

Teacup kids

Children who don't function well without their parents' assistance.

THE
OVERPARENTING
EPIDEMIC

INTRODUCTION

We love our children. We want the best for them—whatever that may be. We want to be sure that they will have every opportunity in this world to succeed—however we may define success. In fact, we often try to do everything we possibly can to *guarantee* that our children will have *every* chance to attain *every* level of success. That means that we want to provide them with the means to match or surpass us—their parents—and the lifestyle they have experienced growing up.

So what might that look like for today's parents? What guarantees our success in raising a new generation of wonderful children, destined to make this world a better place? Because there is no definitive guide, what's a parent to do if he or she wants to do an effective job of raising his or her child? Unfortunately, no university features a Department of Parenting, teaching young adults the skills that they will need to negotiate parenting in the twenty-first century. There's no such thing as student parenting, and nothing that compares to student teaching, which is necessary for anyone pursuing a formal career in education. In the United States, we have no government agencies—on federal, state, or local levels—that require new parents to accrue any knowledge that will help them raise healthy, safe, and responsible children. And because babies don't arrive with an owner's manual, the eventual lessons that we learn as parents often make themselves clear only *after* our experience of raising children occurs.

By the time we are capable of passing on parenting lessons to our children, they are often grown and not so interested in listening to us tell them what we did or didn't do correctly.

Just as our ancestors were left to their own devices to survive a hostile world full of wild animals, severe elements of nature, and a decided lack of vocabulary, we, too, are on our own when it comes to surviving today's hostile world of wild bullies, fatal climate swings, economic stressors, and a persistent overload of information. These issues, along with many others, affect the way in which we parent our children, but because we want the best for them and fear the worst if we don't pull out all the stops, we sometimes succumb to unreasonable and extreme behavior. Despite our best intentions and an understandable desire to do our best for our kids, we can easily succumb to what we call *overparenting*.

For example, some of us have gone to unusually great lengths, including pulling favors to ensure our child's acceptance into a prestigious preschool *before he or she is even conceived.* Hard to believe, but true, and this practice occurs a lot more often than you might imagine. It's almost as if the consultants are in partnership with Cupid, hovering (at least in spirit) over procreating couples, warning them of the pitfalls of conceiving a child without first securing a place for the little one in the best preschool available. This premature hysteria often inspires parents to do whatever it takes (short of committing a crime) to ensure that their children have the "best of the best." This can include enrolling children in what are considered to be exclusive afterschool programs and childhood social activities, making connections for "productive" or "prestigious" playdates, building résumés with questionable facts, hounding coaches for more playing time on the soccer field, securing summer jobs and internships for our teenage children, emailing teachers to procure better grades, hiring consultants to steer acceptance into "top" schools, working the phones to gain employment for kids, helping college freshmen gain admittance into fraternities, choosing unnecessary cosmetic surgeries before a child is fully developed, overscheduling tutors, buying age-inappropriate cars, going on over-the-top vacations, eavesdropping on phone calls, monitoring emails, and placing electronic trackers into teenagers' vehicles.

This is not fiction. When it comes to each and every one of these examples, too many parents are guilty, not just on an occasional basis, but all too often, in every arena, and at every stage of their child's development. Why is it that in today's society the behavior we define as overparenting—as we have just begun to illustrate here—is so often perceived to be ideal? If parents don't already begin over-reaching while their baby is still in the womb, external pressures can begin, in some cases, as soon as a baby is born. Just observe how many audiovisual offerings are on display in stores and online, catering to parents of newborns, baiting them, teasing them with the idea that if their babies watch videos of Einstein, they will improve their chances of attending MIT, or if they start early enough with flashcards (the complete series, of course), they can avoid the humiliation of raising a child who may not read before he or she is out of diapers.

What is going on here? How did what initially seems like support so quickly become pressure and even sabotage? Right from the start, genuine concern can turn into coddling, and keen interest may become infantilizing. We are essentially undermining our children's long-term development, and inhibiting their self-esteem and self-confidence.

It's perfectly understandable that parents want the best for their children. It has been and should continue to be a mantra for all of us. But taking it all too far can become so easily seductive. It begins with parents who are determined that *their* kids will not—under any circumstances—fall short of the lifestyle in which they have grown up. And a top-flight education—no matter what the cost may be—is often viewed as the ticket to make that happen.

Where do these ideas come from? When we see people who practice a certain brand of intensive parenting, we sometimes wonder what prompted such behavior. Where do these overly intense, hyperfocused parents come up with theories to justify their behavior? How did they acquire what they consider to be a sophisticated knowledge of child development, particularly when most of them are probably not childcare experts on any level? Besides the relentlessly steady stream of free advice, which includes the hounding and guilt trips that friends and grandparents seem to supply, there are innumerable child-rearing books, parenting websites, and community seminars, starting with Lamaze classes, all of which are presented by self-appointed experts who promise parents that if they do as prescribed, they will also become parenting experts. Ironically, this book may cure parents of the need to be "experts."

Parents also practice what we might call "selective training for success." This amounts to actively assessing a child's talents, often closely influenced by parents' own preferences and biases, and then directing a diverse schedule of leisure activities while consistently intervening at school and other institutional settings on the child's behalf.

Finally, parents closely monitor many aspects of their children's lives, from their first breaths through their teenage years, sometimes intruding even further into their college careers, and in some cases continuing well into their children's twenties or thirties, as they make every effort to get their children admitted into graduate school and even secure their first jobs.

Many of these behaviors may be well intentioned, but the consequences are often quite negative. Our view is that too much involvement in a child's life can often be destructive, not only for the child but also for the parent. We will demonstrate that position again and again, from one chapter to the next. Hopefully, we will also help you understand how you can fight the impulse to overparent and save yourself from hurting your child—and yourself—in the process.

We can't help asking these questions: What are parents today so afraid of, that they behave so unreasonably and feel justified in doing so? Why do parents think that what they do will make their children perfect—and why do they even think that they should aim for this goal?

"If we never give our children permission to get things wrong," says Jennifer Finney Boylan, professor of English at Colby College and author of *Stuck in the Middle With You: A Memoir of Parenting in Three Genders*, "they're unlikely to ever learn how to get things right."[1] In fact, our children may simply become fearful of risking anything that has not been previously approved by their parents. Do we really want our children living like this—so deeply under our influence that they are not free to discover who *they* are? It's as if our fear of their getting hurt or failing keeps us from allowing them to try things on their own, to learn what they like and dislike and what they can and cannot do.

Children grow up and become adults and then become parents themselves. It's inevitable. It's *The Lion King*, the circle of life, happening right in our backyard, and it's our job as parents to ready our children for leaving the nest, to give them the courage, creativity, and steadfastness to not just survive but flourish out there in what can be a big, bad, scary world, but one that is also undeniably exciting and exhilarating, with limitless possibilities.

Speaking of scary, everyone who is honest is often terrified that they won't be a good—or good enough—parent. If they claim otherwise, they're simply lying or terribly self-centered. By the time we are old enough to have children, most of us are quite set in our ways and may have even started to understand who we are, so it can be shockingly difficult and unsettling to suddenly—overnight, in fact—be faced with having to then help new human beings, especially our own children, develop their own identity and express their unique needs, despite the fact that they have no logical way to communicate those whims and wishes.

As new parents with no previous experience and loads of anxiety, many of us tend to overcompensate. As a result, overparenting can start, as we said, during pregnancy and may intensify with each passing day, as budding mothers and fathers are assaulted with information, telling them what they should and should not do, from how to ensure an optimal pregnancy to laying the foundation for a future member of *Who's Who* or the *Fortune 500*.

Avoid these hazards! Buy this product! Eat meat! Don't eat meat! Exercise like this! Not like that! Drink more! Drink less! Let your baby cry! Do not let your baby cry! There is no shortage of literature pointing out what products to avoid and which foods to buy, what exercises to do, and what books to read, all pointing toward the optimal development of our children. Even during pregnancy, which should be a wonderfully relaxed time of looking forward to a shared future of raising a family, all this advice and needless advertising can turn that joyful, bonding time into a nine-month, anxiety-ridden obstacle course of unnecessary things to buy and risks to be avoided.

Then, as soon as the baby is born, concerns about his or her safety take center stage, and the 24-7 march of monitoring begins. Before we as parents even realize it, we are watching our child's every move— like hawks! Our child doesn't have the opportunity to just experiment and play on his or her own. Every gesture is commented upon, every look becomes a cause for concern or excitement, and every piece of poop is ripe for analysis. When we can't physically be in the same room, we have monitors to alert us to every breath, sound, and move a baby makes. We create the illusion that we are in control and can protect our children from everything! That effort to protect and control is something that all good parents do, but much faster than we realize, this overinvolved behavior can quickly become part of our parental DNA. Some parents who employ a nanny install video equipment, sometimes known as a "nanny cam," to secretly monitor the nanny's behavior. Safety, management, and control are paramount to what is perceived to be good, effective, and possibly even perfect parenting.

This growing obsession among new parents continues as their first baby takes his or her initial steps in the world, announcing his or her developing independence. With those first steps, some parents accelerate their hovering, lurching, ready to pounce at any sign of unsteadiness, making sure that their curious toddler does not walk into a wall or fall down any steps. Naturally, safety is a concern for any parent, as it should be, but many moms and dads are already—and unknowingly—stifling their children's burgeoning autonomy by their somewhat misguided concern for their children's welfare, as if the children might break if they plop to the floor as they attempt to walk. Of course they will fall—over and over again—and gloriously, too. We all do! Each and every one of us experiences failure in the early stages of learning something new. It's natural and to be expected. Learning from our mistakes is the foundation of all education, from our first attempts to get food into our mouths to solving the mysteries of science. Trial and error, the amazing process of learning about the world around us—and ourselves—universally begins at birth and essentially never ends. Along the way, it's messy, chaotic, and sometimes maddeningly frustrating, but everyone, even those born with a silver spoon in their mouths, must experience the struggles that life presents and eventually learn how to overcome life's challenges.

This struggle to survive and cope is what makes us who we are! It's the key to developing as a whole person and discovering the beauty of life. So, why do so many parents think that they can—and should—protect their children from the foibles of failure, particularly in this era? By doing so, they are depriving their children—at any age—of the inevitable satisfaction of figuring out things for themselves. That toddler falling down who grows up as an overprotected child may turn out to be a twenty- or thirty-something-year-old who still hasn't figured out how to fend for himself or herself and still calls his or her parents for help every time something does not go smoothly, which is what happens in life. Do we really need a society of adults with no knack for problem solving and an alarming lack of ability to stand on their own two feet? This kind of overparenting will only mean that there will be more children with little self-confidence and self-esteem because they never really learned how to take care of themselves!

With the deluge of hype coming from Madison Avenue, parenting experts, childhood books, toy manufacturers, and an ever-expanding collection of websites devoted to making sure that you "maximize your child's opportunities" and "get it right," it's no wonder that so many parents today are so stressed and in turn overdoing it, that is, overparenting, by trying too hard, pushing too fast, coming on too strong, and essentially parenting from a place of fear, insecurity, and anxiousness.

Some would argue that overparenting is a class issue, a recent phenomenon only infecting parents with a lethal combination of too much time on their hands and a manic drive to succeed in an ultracompetitive world. Others claim that this is just the first-child phenomenon, when parents take photos of their new baby every five minutes and don't stop until they're forcing their kid to pose on the front steps of their freshman dorm. It's a classic situation, where every first child means an overflowing photo album and video library of every burp, bump, and baseball game, but by the time parents bring a fourth or fifth child into the world, all they might manage is a frantic birth picture and a cellphone grab of their kid's high school graduation. Perhaps. But the behavior that we will sample in this book is not simply defined by income, culture, or education. Much of the science—and inevitably the folly—in overparenting cuts across many of these lines.

It certainly is not a strictly American phenomenon. In China, where up until quite recently the government enforced a one-child-per-family law, it's not surprising that those mothers and fathers tend to focus too much attention on their one and only child. On the other hand, consider a modern Orthodox Jewish family in Israel or America, whose culture encourages large families of at least eight or nine children. It's a wonder that those moms and dads can consistently remember the names of their children. They probably don't have many chances to do anything that could be described as overparenting.

These are challenging times for parents to absorb the physical, emotional, and psychological bumps and bruises of raising children. Many are doing a fantastic job, and we should all learn from them. Others are struggling and just need a bit of guidance and encouragement. But some—too many, in fact—are lost when it comes to giving their children strategies for problem solving, along with the resilience that comes with that, which in turn provides a clear path to maturity. Instead, they offer money, pills, and tutors, and if things don't go the way they want, they either bully or manipulate whoever they perceive to be blocking their path to achieving the result that they are seeking.

There is a better way.

CHAPTER 1: ARE YOU OVERPARENTING?

When I was a child over fifty years ago," Sam says, describing his upbringing in Central New Jersey, "I would show up at home for meals, and the rest of the time was mine either to run around with friends, go to my room and do 'experiments,' or ride my bike to the sports fields across town for pickup games—baseball in spring and summer and football in fall and winter. Occasionally, someone would call my parents to tell them they saw me riding my bike through a red light or report me being up to some kind of mischief, like throwing tomatoes at cars or calling up the drugstore to see if they had Prince Albert in a Can. From what I gather, my childhood was similar to my parents', and their parents', too. It was simple and real and uncomplicated."

Today, in small towns and communities throughout America, in places such as Bainbridge Island near Seattle, Washington, or L'Anse, Michigan, on the Upper Peninsula, or Cape Cod, Massachusetts, kids still live like that. Their parents do not have afterschool programs for their kids. Those children go home after school and play for hours, like kids have been doing for decades, largely unsupervised and left alone to be children, surviving on their own devices and left to think for themselves. That means enjoying the pure pleasure of creating something out of nothing, as well as figuring out for the most part how to deal with mistakes and troubles—on their own, all by themselves. In places like this, where people can live life literally out of the fast lane, parents generally don't fret about their children's welfare, try to manage every activity their kids are engaged in, or continually text them to "check in." Amazing. Kids can be kids—creative, conniving, and cantankerous, yet quite capable of growing up successfully, leaving the adults to pretty much do the same, but hopefully in private. Is it because parents in rural communities have it easier than those trying to navigate life in the big city? Maybe. Maybe not. The grass is always greener, if you want to look at life that way, and it always has been.

When it comes to parenting, we all have our ups and downs, good days and bad days, moments to be proud of and occasions to cringe. Despite our differences—culturally, economically, or by virtue of age, gender, or education—we all share one thing in common: overparenting. We're all guilty. At some point or another, we've all gone overboard trying to do what we consider to be the right thing for our children. While our intentions are almost always admirable regarding our children, our specific actions may prove otherwise.

The traps and foibles of modern-day overparenting are basically unavoidable, especially when you consider one primary object: the cell phone. With this mobile device, we can keep track of our kids at just about any time and any place. And, if they don't respond when we email, text, or call (or all three), it can create terrible anxiety for the parent and make the child feel infantilized and intruded upon, many times for no good reason. It's a great example of when a concern for our children's safety can become a need for control, and as our children get older, this can become quite counterproductive. Overparenting can also come into play because of the great pressure so many parents feel to make sure that they are doing the right thing, so that their children will be successful. This pressure can lead to overscheduling, overpraising, overtutoring, and generally overstressing about life itself.

What we refer to as "overparenting" covers a broad spectrum of parental involvement. At times, all of us may feel the need to intervene, either to help our children when they absolutely need it or to jump in and give our child a leg up on everyone else. Perhaps you don't always recognize the difference, and a definition is required:

Overparenting occurs when someone tries too hard to manage the outcome of his or her child's life, imposing his or her own expectations, often inappropriately, regardless of the child's wishes and abilities.

Sound familiar? Wait, there's more:

Overparenting violates reasonable boundaries when a parent undermines a child's developing independence by sabotaging a teacher or coach's authority or through unnatural attempts to manipulate institutions that might otherwise present healthy and productive life challenges.

In all honestly, we're not quite finished:

Overparenting can compromise a child's ability to deal with hardship and failure, can stunt the growth of self-esteem and confidence, and can lead a child to feel a warped sense of entitlement and unreasonable expectations. Ultimately, this can create a sense of failure on the part of the parent, particularly when his or her efforts to manipulate and scheme for a successful outcome do not work out.

While all of this behavior may not apply to you, some of it must be all too familiar, either through firsthand experience or from behavior you have witnessed. In any case, each of us, no matter how diligent and thoughtful we may be, can hardly avoid the pitfalls and pressures that parenting inevitably presents, which includes the daily possibility of overparenting our most prized possessions: our children.

Time-out! What's wrong with that last sentence? It's quite simple. While at times we may feel that our children are our most prized possessions, they are not actually your possession or your trophy, no more than a spouse is to his or her mate.

Your child is not your possession.

Get that straight right now, because it is crucial to your ability to parent a healthy, happy, and productive citizen of the world. Your child, aside from the person with whom you conceived him or her, is probably the most important, most loved person in your life, and that's a good thing; that's how it should be. But that's where it also needs to stop. This is twenty-first-century America. You don't own your child any more than you own your husband or wife.

You must recognize that while your child is supported by you—a little or a lot, depending on his or her age—an essential part of your job as a parent is to teach your child, beginning with his or her first steps, how to become independent; then, as he or she does achieve this, you must let the child go. But that's difficult for many people, especially those who confuse letting go with not loving their child enough. Maybe it would help if these moms and dads had a simple way to determine their own level of overparenting. It's almost impossible to evaluate our own behavior without a little outside help, an objective eye to clarify our strengths and weaknesses, so we have developed a checklist for you to use to gauge your own behavior.

How Do You Know whether You Are Overparenting?

This brief series of multiple-choice questions will give you a pretty clear estimation of how much overparenting you're doing—or not. Hint: There is no perfect answer! And because there is not always even a "correct" answer that applies to every parent, child and situation, you must determine what's right for you and your family. If you're not sure, keep reading. This book should help you figure some of it out.

1. Do you sacrifice your own social needs simply to attend to your child?

    A. Sometimes.

    B. All the time.

    C. Rarely.

    D. I have no social needs of my own, or, if I do, they revolve around my child's schedule.

2. Are your happiness and self-worth tied up solely in your children?

    A. Sometimes, but isn't that true of all parents?

    B. It depends on what else is going on in my life. Let me check my calendar.

    C. No, absolutely not.

    D. Yes—although it's hard to admit, I am only as happy as my unhappiest child.

3. How often do you do your kid's kindergarten project?

    A. Never.

    B. Usually, especially if it's late at night and it hasn't been done yet.

    C. Always. Aren't we supposed to?

    D. Sometimes. If he asks, I'll supervise.

4. Do you feel bad if your kid's third-grade science project looks inferior to the ones that were done by parents?

    A. Not really.

    B. Of course! It's embarrassing, and people will think I'm a bad parent.

    C. Sometimes, especially if the teacher seems to reward those kids whose parents helped.

    D. No—as long as my kid doesn't care, I'm fine.

5. Whose fault is it if your child is not admitted into his or her college of choice?

   A. The high school—in particular, the guidance counselor.

   B. The college, because it didn't appreciate my child's gifts.

   C. No one is at fault.

   D. The College Board, for making these tests so freaking important!

6. What should happen if your ninth-grade child is struggling academically?

   A. Switch to a different school.

   B. Call the school and demand new teachers.

   C. Encourage your child to speak with his or her teachers.

   D. That's impossible. My kid's a genius, but they are not testing him correctly.

7. How often should you be texting your child during the school day?

   A. Only when I really miss him.

   B. Two or three times, but not during lunch. I want her to eat!

   C. Never.

   D. It's a two-way street with my child. I like him to initiate our daily texting.

8. If your seven-year-old is being bullied on the playground, what will you do first?

   A. Confront the bully's parents after school.

   B. Speak with your child and get his or her account.

   C. Punch out the bully and ask questions later.

   D. Ask the teacher on duty what is happening, why, and how it can be stopped.

9. How much "down" time do you allow your child?
    A. None. The world is competitive, and there's no time for that.
    B. "Down" time means community college instead of an Ivy League school, so none of that.
    C. Here's a stick. Go play in the backyard.
    D. I make sure that my kids have time to relax every single day.

10. What will you do if your child graduates from college and can't get a job?
    A. Call up colleagues and get one for him.
    B. Give him an allowance and tell him not to worry.
    C. Go to his job interviews with him and try to seal the deal.
    D. Offer him ninety days of home therapy.

11. Do you still pay your twenty-six-year-old's cell phone bill?
    A. How else will she get the family plan discount?
    B. It's the only way I know that she will call me.
    C. No. She can talk to whomever she wants on her nickel.
    D. I've been doing it for years. Why would I change a good thing?

A Color Code for Parents

Like the color-coding system that the Transportation Security Administration (TSA) once used to signal specific threat levels of terrorism and announce its responsive course of action, we might also use this system, thanks to the suggestion of a school counselor in Texas, to delineate a spectrum of parental behavior that ranges from absolutely healthy, to not-so-much, to sick, to downright worthy of an urgent visit to the emergency room or psychiatric clinic. Almost every parent, depending on the situation, moves between the green, yellow, orange, and red zones at different times in their child's life. Some parents seem to be always in a crisis mode, and to them everything is seen as a cause for alarm, if not a potential threat to their child's success in the world. In the same manner as the TSA, these colors seem like a reasonable way to evaluate one's level of overparenting, from caring and supportive, to worried and confused, to desperate and out of control.

Green
A parent is confident and caring, and able to foster the development of resilience, independence, and freedom in his or her children.

Yellow
This is when caring becomes controlling, when a worried parent moves in to actively intervene in situations in an effort to affect the outcome.

Orange
As a parent becomes worried, often for no apparent reason, he or she becomes manipulative and even more controlling, trying to take charge of the school, the teachers, and anyone else he or she can reach. At these times, the parent will often be seen as mean if not downright nasty.

Red
This is when a parent's behavior simply gets out of control. While a real crisis may demand an extreme response—for example, when a child's survival is at stake—we all too often see parents reaching this level of behavior when it is *not* warranted. When a parent is out of control, when he or she becomes "crazy," this can create damaging consequences for the child and the relationship with his or her parent.

Your level of overparenting is subject to change based on your anxiety, intelligence, self-control, ability to reason, capacity for discretion, and threat level. There is an extensive history spanning many decades of what degrees of parental involvement and behavior are deemed to be appropriate.

According to *The New York Times*, Diana Baumrind, a clinical and developmental psychologist at the University of California, Berkeley, has found that "the optimal parent is one who is involved and responsive, who sets high expectations but respects her child's autonomy."[1]

Active parents like these define the best aspect of what "controlling" can be, an ideal balance of caring, discipline, and respect. Their children will thrive academically and socially, as opposed to children of parents who are either permissive and less engaged, or controlling and too intense.

It's a challenge to find the best mix, and it depends on many factors. But there are many warning signs to consider that can help you identify whether you might be overparenting.

Parenting Archetypes

In order to fully understand the variety of behavior and personality traits that define the world of overparenting, it is important to identify who these archetypes are, what they do, and *why* they do it. Clearly, we will not list all of them, as not even Shakespeare could include all of society's archetypes in any one play, but the characters that follow should help you identify where you fit in the collection. While some of these archetypes overlap somewhat, we've divided them into five distinct categories: guardian angels, type-As, buddies, producers, and accessories. Please remember that most parents may overlap categories. Just as one size does not fit all, one person may not personify one archetype alone.

GUARDIAN ANGELS

These parents are perpetually hovering nearby, always ready to jump in to protect or facilitate anything that may happen to their children.

The Protector

Who They Are: Like the negotiator and the intervener, these parents are afraid that their children will be hurt, be disappointed, or, even worse, fail at something. With that in mind, they will do almost anything to protect their children from that type of outcome. They will go so far as to lie, manipulate, and cover up for their children so that the children don't have to deal with the consequences of their behavior.

What They Do: A protector will usually just listen to the child's version of whatever incident has occurred, take that story at face value, and then go into defensive or attack mode. At that point, this person will attempt to protect the child from what the parent—and the child—perceive to be the consequences of the child's bad behavior. Even if the child's story is incorrect and offers a distorted view of what happened, which is often the case if the child is "fudging" the facts, the protector will take action. He or she may approach the head of the school and tell that person what the child said, as well as that the teacher is bad, and what the teacher did wrong to cause the child to act inappropriately and to be unfairly subjected to negative consequences. The protector will usually accept the word of the young child over the professional report of the teacher and the school.

Why: If parents have a holier-than-thou attitude about their own position in the world, they may simply avoid digging deeper to understand the position of the school and/or the teacher. They may also mistrust the school or the system with which the child is involved and will quickly blame or find fault with anything having to do with that system. It's often easier to just take the word of the child, assume that he or she is right, and make others fix the problem. Conveniently, this spares the protector, much like the blamer, from holding himself or herself accountable for the child's behavior and his or her own ineffective parenting. It also preserves the child in a positive light, and keeps the child from being upset, which can be very important for parents who choose this behavior.

Example: Alicia, a Midwestern mother of two, has just moved to a new neighborhood and enrolled her kids in the local middle school. Her son, Danny, doesn't like his new school and is lashing out at other kids and his teachers. When his teacher contacts Alicia to describe Danny's behavior, Alicia is deeply embarrassed, and instead of apologizing, looking for solutions, and trying to understand what is happening with her son, she puts on a defensive front and points a finger at the other children and the teacher. The next day, without having discussed any of this with her son, she marches into the school and demands that Danny be moved to another class.

The Hyper-Protector

Who They Are: These parents are seemingly "normal" and begin their parental lives with average concerns for their children's safety, but soon enough they are running interference for their children at every corner, in essence trying to protect them from every potential life risk.

What They Do: Much like interveners and micromanagers, hyper-protectors overreact in many situations, usually before they occur, and then respond by trying to keep their children from participating in typical childhood activities, such as riding school buses, playing in local playgrounds, and enjoying sleepovers, just to name a few.

Why: Hyper-protectors look around at the world, and all they see is its instability and pending dangers. Often this behavior can be triggered by a traumatic event happening to another child or the media picking up on an event involving another child somewhere else, which makes these parents nervous. They may also be trying—unrealistically—to preserve their children's first phase of life, when they were essentially dependent on their parents for everything and their parents reveled in the feeling of being needed.

Example: Mo and Bette live in a suburb of Baltimore, Maryland, which has seen its share of crime over the years. However, Mo and Bette don't live on the set of *The Wire*. Their children attend a private school, and their neighborhood is quite safe. But Mo and Bette cannot relax, and they have hired a driver, who essentially functions as a bodyguard, to escort their children to and from school, as well as to every playdate, sleepover, and sporting event. The "driver" even takes a seat on the daughter's basketball team bench during games. This constant surveillance and watchdogging is causing a terrible rift between Mo and Bette and their children.

The Intervener

Who They Are: They are related to the negotiator, in that they seek to represent their children when conflicts arise with teachers, coaches, or tutors. Unfortunately, they often jump in and make demands without a full understanding of the situation, which includes taking their child's word for what has or has not occurred as it relates to the event for which they are intervening.

What They Do: Much like negotiators, these parents just can't keep their noses out of their children's business. Interveners will often sneak into their children's school to manipulate or pitch for their kids, but they don't want their kids to know that they have tried to intercede. This type of behavior has inspired the term "stealth parent." Even when their kids are upset and tell their parents not to intervene or that they will work it out themselves, these parents do it anyway—because they just can't help themselves, thinking that is what "good parents" do, or because they know that their children will not be able to express themselves as well as the parents do.

Why: These parents often intervene because their kids are "afraid of retribution" if they actively disagree with a teacher or coach about something meaningful to them. Rather than encourage and support their children to stand up and speak for themselves, interveners choose to communicate on their children's behalf, depriving them of the opportunity to become self-confident problem solvers and effective negotiators in their own right, which are life skills they need to develop. This does not necessarily mean that parents should never intervene, but they should give their children the opportunity to try to work it out first on their own.

Example: Dan, a father of three from Lansing, Michigan, is worried about his youngest child, Angel, who loves to play the drums but is not terribly adept at holding a beat. She would like to join her middle school's jazz band someday, but it's quite clear to everyone, Angel included, that she needs much more practice before she's ready to play in public with other students. Angel has a good sense of humor about her struggles, but Dan feels that the school's music teacher should be reaching out to her. In fact, he pressures him to hold an audition for Angel, even though she doesn't want it. This forces both Angel and the music teacher into an awkward and painful situation. Sadly, it's not long before Angel gives up the drums entirely.

The Anxiety Maker

Who They Are: These are the parents we see everywhere, constantly phoning and texting, checking their watches to make sure that they are on time and that they do not miss an activity or contact from anyone about their child. If they have young children, they will be holding their hands everywhere they go, as if a wind is about to blow the children away and they will never be found again.

What They Do: Anxiety-driven parents—most of us can sometimes fall into this category—often do not allow young children to use age-appropriate playground equipment without an adult close enough to physically hold them. Some parents even will put a tracker on their children at a nursery school or another lower school, just in case something happens to them. They will prevent young teenagers from going out with their friends, even to safe places, such as movie theaters or malls, without parental supervision, because the children are "not old enough" or "something might happen." Some parents go so far as to check on their seventeen- or eighteen-year-old children when they are hanging out at a friend's home. Some will even put trackers on their children's cars. They may call and check on them hourly, barrage them with texts, or contact the other child's parents to see what they are up to.

Why: These parents may have high levels of anxiety themselves, and this causes them to overreact, especially when it comes to their kids. Their anxiety often causes their children to become anxious when there is no reason for them to be, and sets up children who may become untrusting of themselves and others, just as their parents are demonstrating with their behavior.

Example: Joan's daughter is in her last year of high school. Joan is in a tizzy, worried that her daughter may not get into the college of her choice. Two or three times a week, she calls the guidance counselor and asks her to remind the prospective colleges about her daughter, but she does not spend nearly as much time ensuring that her daughter is doing her homework, something that will have a more significant impact on her getting into college. Joan is also anxious that her daughter's self-esteem will suffer if she is not selected to be this year's homecoming queen.

TYPE As

These parents are driven in every area of their life. Their home life and involvement with their children is just another part of that.

The Overachiever

Who They Are: The overachiever is typically a highly educated, professionally trained mom who has quit her job and now devotes herself full-time to parenting, focusing like a laser on her only child because she has "just one chance to get it right or make it perfect." This means, based on her own exceptional achievements, which she feels that she has given up to raise her child, she has extremely high expectations for her child's academic outcomes. It becomes particularly trying for the overachiever and her child if the child is not as gifted as the parent feels he is, or at least *should* be.

What They Do: These parents will have their children take standardized tests, such as the PSAT, up to five times so that they will get a better score. These parents are convinced that this type of pushing will give their children a step up on the academic ladder. These parents often want their children to go to the college of *their* choice and direct their children's application process in that direction, not seriously considering what would be a good fit for their children or even what the children may want. When a guidance counselor asks a child of an overachiever where he or she wants to go to college, the answer may often begin with, "My mother thinks I should go to . . ."

Why: These parents are as keen to be successful in parenting as they have been at their work, and their success is measured by their child's performance. They would feel inadequate as a parent if their child fell short in any of the endeavors they deem important, whether those are in the classroom, on the field, or in a concert hall. They assume, and possibly even announce, that their child is special and more intelligent than other children, and because of that, they push their child all the time to make sure that their claims will not be proven wrong. Because they chose to back out of their careers, which they later view as "their sacrifice," these parents obviously have a hole to fill in their lives, and they all too often mistakenly try to fill it by placing unreasonable expectations on their children.

Example: Mimi, a self-acknowledged helicopter parent, is very well educated and was a successful business executive until she stopped working to take care of Cindy, her only child. She immediately began managing all of her daughter's activities, scheduling her life as if she were her supervisor instead of her mother. It wasn't long before Mimi became supercritical of Cindy's first teacher and tore her apart at a teacher-parent conference—in front of Cindy. In the absence of her own career challenges, Mimi is running Cindy's life as if she were a small company.

The Controller

Who They Are: Close relatives to the micromanagers, these parents often admit that they are "control freaks" and are proud of it, and may not necessarily see that as being a bad thing when it comes to focusing on their children.

What They Do: When their children are faced with choices, these parents tell their children what to do rather than guide and teach them ways to cope and choose. They insist on making most of the decisions related to their child, such as school subjects, clothing, friends, essay subjects, and which college to apply to and attend. In some cases, this need for control can lead to parents' restricting their children's activities, friendships, and modes of travel. Even when their children are quite young, controlling parents give them constant instructions, even in public places, but often from afar, rather than up close, which further ensures the child's cooperation. In other words, the children are hearing, "Don't touch that," or "Sit down," or "Move away from that lady," or "Don't touch that" (again and again).

Why: Why are control freaks control freaks? Good question. Some people have trouble trusting themselves, and consequently they are not able to trust their own children or most other people in their lives. Others may have previously experienced an especially upsetting event or loss, which led them to decide that if they could manage every aspect of their life, they would never have such an upsetting thing happen again. Others become control freaks with their own children because their parents neglected them during their childhood. As a result, they want to try to undo the fallout of that experience by being a superparent. Naturally, they often overcompensate.

Example: Diane, a ninth-grade parent from New York City, demands a meeting with everyone at school—teachers, administrators, and specialists—because according to daily reports posted online, her daughter is not doing her homework. Diane brings her daughter's tutor to join the twelve teachers and staff in attendance. While the tutor presents the entire agenda, holding the school accountable rather than Diane's daughter, Diane says nothing. Neither does her daughter, who is learning fast that if she doesn't do her homework, Mom will save her. This is an excellent example of underparenting your child and overparenting your school.

The Negotiator

Who They Are: Not surprisingly, these parents consider everything in their lives—and the lives of their children—to be negotiable. That means that they are afraid or unwilling to let their children deal with a difficult situation or the consequences of their behavior on their own. As a result, they will negotiate for their children, thinking that they are helping them.

What They Do: Parents visit school offices, often without an appointment, to try to negotiate a change in their child's schedule, to select a new teacher, to negotiate a higher grade, or even to influence the recommendation that a teacher will write for the child. By placing such demands on educational institutions, they compromise the ability of the administrators and teachers to do their jobs effectively. This behavior also gives their child the idea that there are no absolutes and that rules are meant to be broken. These parents act as if whatever they want for their child is obtainable by their negotiation, and this gives the child a sense that the parent is all-powerful. This undermines the child's ability and incentive to learn to do things and take care of things for himself or herself.

Why: This behavior occurs regularly, and is not necessarily precipitated by a complaint from the child. Parents may intervene simply because they are unhappy or feel that their child's situation needs improvement. They consider it to be their obligation—if not their right—to smooth the way through for their child and deliver optimal results.

Example: Jane, an ambitious entrepreneur in the deep South, makes a habit of confronting her child's teachers about their homework assignments, complaining that they take too long and don't leave enough time for social obligations. She offers excuses, tries to elicit sympathy, and often ends up demanding concessions from the teachers, even though her child clearly has no serious health issues or a demanding family situation that is preventing the work from being completed. When a teacher doesn't agree to Joan's demands, Joan goes straight to the office to solicit cooperation from the principal.

The Micromanager

Who They Are: Micromanagers are parents who are too involved with their children's lives and can't let them deal with problems they have at school, with sports, or in any other aspect of their lives. They feel that if they prop up their child every step of the way, be it in sports, theater, or academics, he or she will never flirt with failure or experience anything short of achieving an optimal and constant level of success. The only way to guarantee that is to micromanage every aspect of the child's life.

What They Do: They tend to not let their children stumble and fall or get confused or frustrated about *anything*. As a result, they micromanage everything, including their child's behavior, activities, and choice of friends.

Why: They can't bear yielding control of every outcome of their child's life situations. Micromanagers are fearful that if they do not determine every outcome, it most certainly will have bad consequences for their child. It's as if they don't trust themselves, first of all, and therefore they cannot fully trust their children to make good choices that produce healthy and positive outcomes.

Example: Samantha, a stay-at-home mom from Tampa, Florida, is upset because her eight-year-old son is having trouble in school and has not been testing as well as he has in the past. When his first-term report card arrives at home with less than optimal grades, Samantha immediately calls the school principal, jumping over her son's teacher to lodge her complaint and see what will be done about the problem. She initially attempts to scapegoat the teacher rather than explore any other reason for her son's struggles.

While this may not demonstrate micromanaging in its classic form, it is a good example of parents' trying to manage their families like they might manage an office, challenging the top person right off the bat rather than pulling back and conferencing with the person who knows their child best.

In this case, it turned out that Samantha's son needed glasses, and once he adapted to wearing them every day, his grades improved and his mother relaxed—at least for the time being.

BUDDIES

These parents want to be their child's best friend, if not a co-child with their own kid.

The Best-Friender

Who They Are: These are parents who often do not have enough going on in their own lives, crave the companionship of their children, and may see themselves as their children's best friends and pals rather than their parents.

What They Do: These parents constantly inject themselves into their children's daily activities at school and in the rest of their lives so that they can remain a steady presence in all of their child's interactions.

Why: Because they feel unappreciated and left out when their children do not share everything with them, it's probably safe to say that these parents are lacking a challenging career and/or a fulfilling social life of their own. Besides what's lacking in their own lives, they feel that if they are their children's best pals, they will have a better understanding of their children and can always be in place to intervene effectively on their behalf. Then, they hope that their children will be grateful and acknowledge their wonderfulness, thereby validating the parents as a worthwhile part of their lives. Being a buddy means that one doesn't have to be a parent who makes hard decisions that the child may get upset about. Instead, these parents hope that they can talk their children into something by being their "pals."

Example: Sylvia has two daughters, one twelve and the other fifteen. When each of them first created a Facebook page, Sylvia insisted that they "friend" her so that she could monitor their activity. Her kids understood the situation, but now that they are both older, they wish that their mother would stop constantly "liking" everything they post and refrain from posting almost daily pictures of them as little girls.

The Assister

Who They Are: These parents are a variation on the protector, as they will go to any length—at any time—to help their child avoid dealing with any unhappiness or troubling life situations. They are ready to rush in and help, no matter what the request is or how inconsequential it may be.

What They Do: Assisters will drop whatever they are doing and rush to school simply because their children call, asking the parents to deliver something that the children have forgotten, whether it's lunch, a homework assignment, or a soccer uniform.

Why: This behavior could be motivated by parents' fear that they will become irrelevant in the lives of their children or that they will have to deal with reality and hardships, in many cases exceedingly minor ones. Too many parents do not have lives of their own. They are seeking to be "buddies" with their children in ways that are unrealistic and unhealthy for both parties.

Example: Chris is a real-estate agent with one child in the seventh grade of a large public school. Chris makes a habit of stopping by the school every afternoon to check her daughter's locker and make sure that she has what she needs. Sometimes, if her daughter has rushed out in the morning without her lunch, Chris will drive over and knock on her daughter's classroom door and stand outside, waving it to get her attention. In the evenings, Chris always helps out with her daughter's homework, to the point of often completing it for her. "We did it!" she says, as if it were supposed to be a team effort.

The Spoiler

Who They Are: These parents consistently do too much for their children—at any age. To make matters worse, they often expect other adults to also indulge their children and will try to shame them when they don't. The spoiler buys expensive presents for their children or takes them on exotic trips without any regard for teaching them the value of work, commerce, and consumerism. Once a trip has been planned, even if the child misbehaves, the parent often feels obligated to go on the trip with the child, further ignoring the idea of teaching a child the consequences of his or her behavior.

What They Do: Spoilers will do just about anything to accommodate their children, eager almost beyond reason to make their lives as easy and pleasurable as possible. They don't want their children to feel frustrated or hurt in any way, much less delay any aspect of their gratification. This sounds OK. We want the best for our kids, but what happens when a child has to survive in the real world, beginning with the daily culture of a kindergarten class? Is it any wonder that early education specialists have to spend almost as much time minding parents as they do them.

Why: Reasons vary, but parents who are extremely busy and focused on their own business and social lives don't often spend significant time with their children. To assuage their guilt, they treat their children with expensive presents or trips instead of spending time and actually doing things with them. What this usually adds up to for the child is a crowded closet and an empty heart.

In other cases, spoilers, who may have missed something in their own lives growing up, try to overprovide what they did not get. This can also become a way to control their children by giving them things, which in turn helps the parents feel needed and worthwhile. With older kids this takes the form of buying them things that they could not afford on their own and continues their dependence on their parents. This approach often backfires, as children grow up feeling entitled and may flaunt their stuff as a way to gain acceptance, but, in fact, this serves to distance them from their peers, and may well stunt the natural growth of their independence.

Example: "I wake my son up three times every day to make him get out of bed," says Ingrid, a Swedish mom of a university student. "I wash his clothes and cook all his meals. I feel like I am needed and that is nice—to feel important. I'm not sure how that's working for my son, but it makes me feel good."

The Smotherer

Who They Are: These parents take the archetype of best-friender to another level. They try to constantly be with their children. If they could attend school, sleepovers, and every school trip with them, they would, no matter how old their children may be. They are the ones who insist on being chaperones on school trips, volunteers in the library, and monitors at school dances. As their kids get older, this becomes a major cringe moment for them.

What They Do: Teachers report that they've seen parents become far too involved in their children's play and friends, especially when there is even a mild dispute. When these teachers tried to encourage the students to work things out themselves without involving their parents, the children told them that their parents would decide what they should do. Some parents have been known to come to school, find the other child, and have a word with him or her.

Smothering parents are also known to sit in public places with their adolescent children and maintain constant monitoring, not leaving the children with any anonymity or lack of supervision.

Why: For some reason, these parents do not trust their children to be their own people, as if they couldn't possibly be autonomous without the involvement of their parents. They may feel that they did not do a good enough job raising their children so that the children would have internalized their values, and that without their input the children would be unable to navigate on their own.

Example: A Montessori school in the Northeast that we've observed is typical of most schools. It has a strong parent base of volunteers for academic and nonacademic programs. In fact, the willingness of the parents to get involved became a problem last year when the school had no choice but to cancel a field trip because too many parents volunteered to chaperone. The school could not accommodate such a large number of chaperones, and because no parent agreed to withdraw, it was cancelled.

PRODUCERS

These parents view their children as products that they are turning out into the world.

The Consumer

Who They Are: These parents are usually found in private school settings, where they equate everything about their children's "success" with the fact that they have picked the school, are paying the school, and have clear expectations about what results they expect for their money.

What They Do: For these parents, creating the "perfect" child means choosing (or using a consultant to choose) and then paying for what they perceive to be the best approach to produce the outcome they want for their child. Then, they expect the school to do it all from there, which means that the parents should have immediate and unfettered access to the school director, and to the teachers who are supposed to make it easy for their child, independent of the child's input or effort, because in their view the results should be equivalent to the money they have spent on tuition. This becomes an even bigger issue if they become board members of the school, where they feel as if they can demand anything, at any time, including no consequences for their child's bad behavior.

Why: Over the past two decades, there has been a huge shift in parental entitlement, and it's not only prevalent in the private school sector. It is happening everywhere. Public school parents, aware that, as taxpayers, they are paying the salaries of their children's teachers, may make unreasonable demands beyond the normal range of professional and ethical accountability. Lower-income families may push hard to get their children into a charter school and then try to equate their children's success with the value of their vouchers. This consumer mentality on the part of the parents may be caused in part by an erosion of school authority as well as the hyped-up demands of our ever-intensifying consumer society. This can cause a considerable lack of respect for school administrators and teachers. In fact, there seems to be a view today that education is just another commodity and that a parent should be able to make demands, however outrageous they may be, of the product that is offered and the results it produces. Unfortunately, this leaves out an essential human element and does not allow for the ups and downs of child development.

Example: A private school director from southern Connecticut has heard the following on numerous occasions:

"I am paying good money for my kid's education, and I want you to take care of everything he needs and be accountable for what I paid for. That also means that I should be able to call the school and have you answer me whenever, and for whatever I want."

"These parents are essentially referring to their children as 'my product,' which is a strange way to think about your child, unless you view the whole process from a consumer's angle. Consumerism is dangerous because of parents who donate money to the school beyond tuition costs and then think that their kids—and they—should get special privileges. Like, even when their kids get into trouble and should deal with the consequences, the parents say, 'You have no loyalty,' as if donating money should get them special treatment."

Example: A parent and school board member was upset when her child was not allowed to play in a football game because he had previously failed a test. The parent called up the headmaster, pointed out how the family had been at the school for two generations, the son was a full-fee student, and, as a board member, she had paid a lot of money and had a significant amount of clout to affect the principal's job, particularly if her son did not get to play.

The Blamer

Who They Are: These parents are unwilling to let their children experience unpleasant consequences as a result of their actions and tend to be unwilling to look at their own parenting as one of the reasons why their children got into difficulty in the first place. Instead, they blame everyone else except themselves and their own children for most if not all of the problems that arise.

What They Do: They will fight for their children to have what they want rather than tough it out and face the appropriate consequences for their behavior. This means that the children do not have the opportunity to learn from their mistakes and be able to move on and do better, when and if the situation arises again. Depriving children of the chance to face difficulties on their own will not do the children any good. Their first response will probably be to get mad at their parents for trying to "help."

Why: As parents, we all want to control the environment we live in, hoping to create the most pleasant circumstances possible for our children. However, the real world is not always so kind or forgiving or accepting, and we cannot control it anywhere near as much as we would like——for ourselves or our kids. To say, "My kid should never be frustrated or confused" may be a fine sentiment, but it's not terribly realistic. So when a child becomes frustrated or confused, the best thing we might do for them is have them look first in the mirror and ask "Why" because in many cases they themselves are at least partially responsible for their predicament.

Example: A public high school administrator describes a chronic problem of parents' jumping into a conflict without knowing the full story of their children's behavior:

"One of our students was caught smoking cigarettes in the bathroom. Naturally, a teacher had him sent to me. He tried to excuse himself by complaining about how stressed he was at school and how smoking was his only relief. When I pointed out that it was simply against the rules of the school—for everyone—he blamed our school for making his life so difficult. As soon as we finished our conversation, with his emotions still high, he called his mom and gave her his slant on our conversation. Not two minutes later, she called me, expressing her deep concern and frustration about what had been discussed with her son. As is too often the case, this parent was blaming our school for her son's problem before even asking for my objective side of the story."

Besides getting the facts wrong because she bought into her son's apparent lies, this parent was blaming the wrong person. In fact, she was making excuses for him instead of seeking the truth and holding him accountable for his actions. Perhaps the mother was also a smoker and felt as if the school was indicting her as well as her son.

The Delegator

Who They Are: These are often overly busy parents (see consumers) who view their child as just one of the many projects they are responsible for in their lives. They expect all the big issues to be dealt with by someone else, be it the school, the nanny, the coach, or the tutor. It's as if they imagine that they can actually outsource their role as parents.

What They Do: They delegate nearly all responsibility for their child to schools, athletic teams, tutors, and babysitters. Some refer to this as "absentee parenting" or "outsourced parenting."

Why: These parents have other priorities, such as work, golf, social obligations, and indulgences, which supersede being directly involved in their child's life. If they were asked, they would say that their child is important to them, but in reality, they think that the other things that they are doing are just as valuable, if not more so. This may be caused by something that happened in their childhood, for example, having neglectful parents of their own, or because of unusual demands they are experiencing at work. For others, it is simply that they are self-centered and cannot put someone else first, not even their own children.

Example: Norris is a high-powered lawyer with a teenage son, who he sees as a candidate to take over his law firm in the future. He has put together a staff of drivers, tutors, and trainers to make sure that his son is never late to school or any extracurricular activity (of which there are many) and has hired a personal assistant to submit weekly reports on his son's productivity.

The Disrespecter

Who They Are: These parents are a variation on the blamer and the consumer and have a tendency to act badly toward the people who are most responsible for raising their children. They tend to view themselves as high-status people, and therefore all the people they hire or who work for them, from their children's teachers to nannies to coaches, are treated as people who do not know what they are doing or are not doing it well enough. Subsequently, the parents criticize these other people to the point of disrespect, rather than appreciating what they do for their children and their families as a whole.

What They Do: These parents tend to view no one as being as important or as wise as they are, and instead of looking at the big picture, they focus on every reason they can find for why things are not going as they expected for their child. Rather than looking for what they can do to make the situation better, or how they can work together with others to improve things, they focus on the shortcomings of everyone else, which leads to disrespectful behavior directed at teachers, school staff, tutors, coaches, and nannies. When children observe this behavior, it can encourage them to also disrespect authority and the roles that these other important adults play in their lives.

Why: Simply put, many of these parents are self-centered, if not downright narcissistic, which may come across as a superiority complex. This behavior is often driven by ignorance, as these parents often have little to no firsthand knowledge of what a teacher does in the classroom, what is involved in being a full-time nanny, or how complex and challenging it can be to coach child athletes, especially those with type-A personality parents.

Example: "I am *paying* you! Therefore, I can disrespect you." What goes without saying is that "I know more than you, even though I have never done what you are doing."

In fact, when parents adopt this stance toward anyone playing a role in their child's life, they are essentially disrespecting their child.

ACCESSORIES

These parents view their children as so important that anything they do in life is just to enhance or embellish their children's lives and activities.

The Cheerleader

Who They Are: These parents can be seen at every school play, after-school activity, science fair, soccer game, and car wash. They're the ones endlessly applauding, heaping praise, and cheering the loudest, particularly for their child. These parents even carry around a daily calendar of their *children's* schedule, not their own, because everything in their life revolves around their children. (Some might call these parents "accessorizers," as they essentially become an accessory to their child's life.)

What They Do: Modern-day cheerleaders go to almost every function that involves their child, both in and out of school, seven days a week, year-round. They become an accessory in their child's life. Some parents may even wear matching clothing and attempt to incorporate their children's jargon into their natural speech. In the "olden days," parents rarely attended their kid's activities and wouldn't be caught dead copying their clothing habits.

Why: Are parents afraid that they will miss something? Could the same syndrome that drives parents of newborns to photograph every other breath their baby takes be causing cheerleaders to scramble their schedules to accommodate *everything* their child is doing? Or are parents simply afraid of feeling guilty if they should miss a game or two, especially if their absence would be pointed out by an overzealous parent who can't help noticing when another parent misses an event. Often these parents did not have the opportunity as children to excel at similar activities, or the child is fulfilling a vicarious wish of theirs. They may bask in the child's activities, and in a reverse manner, hope that the child's prowess will rub off on them and make them seem cooler because they have a child who is engaged in a cool activity.

Example: Simon and Dee used to play soccer in college. Now that their two boys are old enough to play youth soccer, they have thrown themselves into the mix of a hectic schedule of weekend competition and weekday practices in their New England suburban community. Simon and Dee, who own a gardening service, attend each and every practice and game—or at least one of them does. They not only create a large presence by cheering on their boys; they also make a habit of steadily sharing their opinions about soccer—and their boys' prowess—with the coach. This endears Simon and Dee to each other, but the charm just about stops right there. The coach tolerates it because Simon and Dee bought the team uniforms, but their boys are beginning to get harassed by some of the other kids on the team, who think that they should get to play as much as Simon and Dee's sons do.

The Carpooler

Who They Are: These parents drop off and pick up their children every day from school.

What They Do: They meet for coffee after dropping off their kids at school in the morning or assemble in the long line outside of school anywhere from fifteen to thirty minutes before the closing bell. In warmer climates, parents leave their cars and gather together to discuss the current state of the school, which includes gossiping about teachers, administrators, grades, and sports. These conversations invariably lead to teachers being judged (often unfairly) and even blackballed, rumors about school personnel, and some children being scapegoated, particularly those whose parents are not active in the carpool zone.

Why: This usually occurs when parents have too much free time and not enough other interests in their lives.

Example: Melody and Bill meet in their cars every school day afternoon outside their children's elementary school. Melody, a stay-at-home mom who runs a graphic arts business from her living room, is anxious about her daughter's progress in reading and writing. Bill, a single father with his own contracting business, feels the same way about his daughter's first-grade experience. "Why aren't our kids doing better?" they both ask. (For the record, it's October.) Soon, they agree that it must be the teacher's fault. They talk up their theory with other parents, and before long their children's teacher is being raked over the coals in a PTA meeting—unnecessarily—because the children are not yet reading and writing at an acceptable level. Sadly, the bullying does not stop, and the teacher—a reading specialist and district mentor— resigns.

The Trophy Giver

Who They Are: These parents will admit that all children are different, with varying abilities and passions, but feel that all children deserve equal treatment, especially when it comes to recognition and awards. These parents want their children to be involved in a lot of activities and to be good in what *they* want them to be good at, but they want them to be appreciated even if they do not particularly excel at an activity. In essence, they don't want anyone's feelings to be hurt, although even the kids themselves know who is good and who is bad at any activity. But these parents insist that everyone should get a trophy, even if they don't do anything but show up.

What They Do: These parents push for their kids to be in sports or onstage, engaged in theater and/or music projects, as well as anything else that comes along. Then they expect their children to be "winners," with the requisite trophies and prizes, no matter how good or bad their performance may have been. If it has been clearly poor or lacking "championship" form, parents will want to spare their children any hurt feelings or threats to their self-esteem. No matter what, their children must be acknowledged!

Why: Some parents are still trying to re-create their own childhoods by seeking the trophies they did not get when they were kids, or are trying to make up for their own hurt feelings when they did not get something they wanted. Others are living vicariously through their children, whom, again, they are trying to protect from the hurt feelings that come from reality and life. In either instance, they are not giving their children a realistic view of the world and the opportunity to accept their own shortcomings, appreciate the strengths of others, make choices in what they want to do, and develop their own positive self-esteem.

Example: Benjy is nine years old and plays soccer in a large suburban community. He's not on the A-team or even the B-team, and is essentially a benchwarmer on the C-team. But he's content to be part of a team and enjoys the outdoor exercise and camaraderie. At the end of the season he receives a trophy at the team banquet. On the way home, Benjy is perfectly happy, until his parents ask him how it must feel to earn his very own trophy.

"Uh, I don't know. I left the trophy there. What do I need it for?"

His parents are aghast and turn the car around to go back and retrieve the trophy.

"I don't want the stupid trophy!" Benjy says, laughing. "I suck at soccer."

"Benjy!" his father snaps. "You do not suck. Don't you dare say that. You earned that trophy, just like every other boy on the team."

"That's right, Benjy," his mother adds. "You're a wonderful soccer player."

"It's OK, Mom," says Benjy. "Don't worry, Dad. You can have my trophy."

The Maturity Killer

Who They Are: These are the parents who ignore developmental changes in their children, treat them effectively as babies or as if they were younger than they are, and do not encourage a proper process of maturity. (See smotherers and protectors.)

What They Do: These parents carry a five-year-old instead of having him walk, cut up a ten-year-old's food in a public restaurant, do not allow their sixteen-year-old to get a learner's permit to even *begin* to get driving experience, forbid their high-school-age children from watching *Saturday Night Live*, and cook all meals for their twenty-five-year-old son who still lives at home.

Why: In the guise of protecting their children from the real world, these parents are determined to keep their children from becoming independent, successful adults. This may keep them "in the fold" where they can be controlled, and that is usually because these parents do not have faith in their own children, which may indicate that the parents do not have any confidence in their own ability to parent appropriately.

Example: Cynthia is a mother of nine living in Salt Lake City, Utah, and her story is inspiring in a good way. Seven of her children have left home to serve on Mormon Church missions. She has had to let go of each one of her children as they venture out into the world on their own.

"It's easy to spoil your children," she says, "and hold on to them beyond the right time, but in the end it's not healthy for them. It stunts their growth! They must experience the world on their own. As the saying goes, that's the circle of life."

Hands On/Hands Off

It should be clear from examining these archetypes that parenting is complicated but that separating ourselves from our children is vital, as is recognizing that, from an early age, they are independent beings. Despite how many of us act and what many of us may think, our children are *not* extensions of ourselves. Each of them is his or her own person, no matter what stage of development the individual is at. This means that children need to be given the space to try out things and experience failure as well as success. That should begin at any early age, certainly by the time they go to school.

But many parents have a hard time accepting that growth in life involves struggling and that their children's trials and tribulations, including the experience of failure, are an intrinsic part of the process of learning to succeed in life.

Morgan, a stay-at-home, first-time mother, had separation issues motivated by the anxiety she felt about her daughter starting school. When Morgan's daughter began kindergarten, Morgan accompanied her to school, like most parents do. During the first week or two, she joined a handful of other parents who lingered in the classroom for the first thirty or forty minutes. But while the other parents eventually learned to take leave of their children at appropriate times, Morgan's separation anxiety made her stay longer and longer. She tried to laugh it off, telling the other parents that she was just so worried that her "clumsy" daughter might fall or bump into something and get hurt. Quite unremarkably to everyone but Morgan, her daughter was fine and so easily engaged in the minute-to-minute activities that she didn't seem to notice her mother hanging around and fretting. Finally, after weeks of tolerating her presence, the teacher confronted Morgan and suggested that she leave her daughter—and the other children—some breathing room. Morgan broke down in tears and admitted to the teacher that not only did she have nothing to do all day at home without her daughter, but she also couldn't stop worrying that something could happen outside her watch. She went on to admit that her mother had also had separation anxiety when Morgan was first left at school.

For many parents, letting their children go out into the world goes against the grain of what they have been led to believe is successful parenting. Today, an entire profit-driven industry exists that is essentially scaring parents into "doing whatever it takes" to guarantee that their child enjoys every possible advantage. As a result, this raises parents' stress levels, creates unreasonable expectations for their children, and makes their children anxious as well. This, in turn, makes it hard for children to learn how to relax and be themselves. Morgan is well on her way to becoming a shining example of a parent who can't let go.

Less Protection, More Communication

If parents want their children to grow up to become independent, confident adults, they need to practice a bit of what we like to call "benign neglect." It requires a simple attitude adjustment—an easing of the mind and a pulling back on the reins of parental control. That begins with allowing your child to experience a certain amount of frustration and to discover that he can recognize a problem and then fix it by himself, without your active and intrusive intervention. It extends to allowing siblings to fight with each other as they are naturally inclined to at times, and then resolve it on their own. You'll be better off—as will they—if you don't intervene all of the time. Let them work things out. As long as there is no one bleeding, it's probably OK.

But if you can't help yourself—if you suspect that you are being excessively protective, fearful, and inhibiting—try confirming your doubts by asking another parent for an opinion, particularly one who has had several children who seem to be doing well. Reality checks are good! You're not obligated to follow the advice, but seeking it will help you make a better decision on your own.

With that conversation in mind, you may be better equipped to first observe and then communicate with your child. Start with a simple question and then *listen* to his or her answer. Depending on the age and personality of your kid, you may not get much. That's OK. You gave the child a chance, and that's what's important. You can explain your concerns, whether they are for your child's safety, grades, or choice of friends. As long as those concerns are not presented as an indictment and do not reek of any automatic lack of trust in your child's competence, you can engage in an open discussion, exploring the situation and offering whatever advice you deem necessary. But the key is listening to your kid!

Surely you know your child better than most anyone else and are the best judge of what activities are acceptable in terms of safety and what behavior is allowed. What is safe and acceptable will always be a bone of contention between parents and children, but the important thing is for parents to realize that sometimes they just need to let go and get a life.

CHAPTER 2: WHY TWENTY-FIRST-CENTURY PARENTING SEEMS SO HARD

When Ben was eight years old, growing up in Burlington, Vermont, his favorite thing to do was to meet his friends and disappear into the woods to go mud sliding through trails that snaked between the trees. They would spend hours there unsupervised, getting completely filthy and having the best time. When Ben was asked what made that memory so sweet, he said, "Because my parents didn't know where I was."

That was then, and this is now. Ben is now the father of two boys, and he and his wife would never let their kids do what he did: disappear for an entire afternoon into the woods with friends, some of whom his parents didn't even know, and then come back home with three inches of mud caked all over him. Today, his kids would be sent into the woods with requisite survival gear, such as tick repellent, an EpiPen, goggles, extra socks, water repellant boots, an expedition vest with enough pockets to hold supplies for an expedition up Mt. Everest, a GPS tracking device, and a video camera strapped to a high-tech forest exploration helmet.

"My kids never leave the house," says Ben. "They're too busy with their computer games." Ben is kidding, but his point is well taken. For the most part, kids today don't experience the purest of freedoms that their parents and grandparents enjoyed "back in the day." They are certainly privy to things that previous generations didn't have, such as science camps and computer games (the educational ones, of course) and an array of supervised team sports, but much of what they do through their teenage years is manufactured—and managed—by their parents or other adults. Too many kids today, in spite of continual advances in technology, communication, and access to unlimited information, have not experienced the excitement of tempting fate, risking conflict, and rallying together after a round of unexpected difficulty or failure. We can dream about returning our children to the simpler lives of yesterday, but in lieu of actually doing so, we should recognize what is missing and not only allow them to go mud sliding alone in the woods but even encourage it.

What to Expect When Everyone Is Telling You What to Expect

Nobody becomes a parent with a clear understanding of what it really means or involves. Once you figure it out and know what you're doing, your kids are gone, or you have so many by then that you're too tired and distracted to get anything right, and all you really care about is your next nap.

Parents today face unprecedented challenges in raising their children. Most of them seem to be trapped by unreasonable if not unrealistic expectations. But before anyone can attempt to remedy that situation, it is important to recognize the pressures that parents must cope with in today's world.

Each and every day, from the time we wake up and turn on the radio, or check the news online or on TV, we are confronted by an onslaught of mass media communication that is designed to get our attention, primarily by frightening us. This creates feelings of inadequacy, as if we are lacking in at least one of life's most essential qualities. It can translate into perceiving ourselves as fashion-deprived, out of shape, undereducated, or close to financial failure. Even worse, we may be driven to feel unable to care for our family. However we may identify our individual shortcomings, Madison Avenue has somehow succeeded in shaping our needs, perverting our desires, and refocusing our goals. This mind-set invariably infects our entire family, and as parents it affects how we view and raise our children.

When our aspirations and fears are heightened by the relentless noise of mass media, where are we to turn for a reality check? Our neighbors and communities can make our developing neurosis even worse, because peer pressure can create even more distorted expectations. It's so easy for parents to compare themselves to other parents, and in no time, they will think that they should do the same things with their children. What kind of job does that father have? Which car is that mother driving? Where does our neighbor's kid go to school? How do they have the time to coach their kids' sports teams? It's like taking "keeping up with the Joneses" to another level, where, sadly, no one can ever really measure up and there's always a feeling of coming up short—as parents and families as a whole.

Society creates an inordinate amount of pressure to succeed at every level and at all costs. Speaking of costs, the current state of our economy makes parents worry even more about their children's future and makes them put ridiculous premiums on the quality of their children's education. Does the sticker price of a prestigious private school guarantee anything in today's competitive world?

It's enough to make parents recoil and to make any child sick. It actually comes down to an omnipresent fear of failure and a gnawing concern that your child will not make it, and that it will be your fault. Insecurity, anxiety, and a basic lack of trust in existing systems seems to be permeating every facet of our educational system and collective family life. These emotional deficits are caused in good part by people's financial concerns. Families struggling with money problems fear for their future and that of their children. Those with plenty of cash feel a burning desire for more. For the majority somewhere in the middle, the cost of having a family seems daunting. Pregnancy is expensive, made more so by fertility treatments. Adoption is costly and time-consuming, and may come after a series of costly in-vitro fertilization treatments. A surrogate is no less expensive and can involve complicated legal issues. When a person adds on the basic costs for a nanny, extra childcare, private schools, extracurricular activities, specialized summer camps, tutors, and college consultants, it is overwhelming before you even get to the rising costs of college tuition. These days, even community colleges and state universities are becoming expensive, let alone four-year, private liberal arts colleges.

How Did Overparenting Begin?

It is virtually impossible to single out any one central factor when trying to determine why parents have come to be so intensely concerned with every aspect of their children's lives. When did every trace of "live and let live" virtually disappear from our parental vocabulary? Overparenting has existed pretty much since parenting itself. If God was supposedly the father of Adam and Eve, can't we safely say with some confidence that there was clearly some overparenting going on there in the Garden of Eden?

Overparenting apparently ebbed and flowed over the past thousands of years, but it clearly exploded during the 1990s. It was as if the public trust had been damaged enough that it was affecting the very core of our family structures. We had peace and prosperity at home, at least for a majority of people, yet anxiety and fear were permeating our society more and more. While crime rates were going down, parents were ratcheting up their safety measures, keeping their kids within earshot and under constant supervision.

Our country's innocence and general trust in authority was shattered in the 1960s with the assassinations of JFK, Martin Luther King, Jr., and Bobby Kennedy. Our communal belief that governmental institutions would take care of us and protect us continued to erode with the awful realities of the Vietnam War, especially as people came to the conclusion that the military could not be trusted or, even worse, that they might not know what they were doing. This was compounded when Nixon imploded right before our eyes. Collectively, these events created lasting feelings of insecurity as we lost our respect for, reverence for, and belief in our government.

The insecurities and polarization that we have come to feel as a nation have bled into our personal behavior and have seemingly gotten worse. While many parenting authorities feel that the rash of overparenting that we have seen since the 1990s is past its height, we disagree. As evidenced here, we can see that parents are as tightly wound as ever, and the prognosis for their children is troubling. Perhaps an examination of human behavior over the ages will help us understand where we are today and put us on the road to being better parents. It is important to note that being a better parent is different from overparenting.

A Brief History of Parenting

Parental involvement in children's lives has changed dramatically throughout history. Whether you subscribe to creationism, take stock in the science of evolution, or lean toward a different vision of history, it's informative to see how parenting has developed and changed since the first baby was born.

Stone Age parents were not exactly diligent when it came to their children's dental hygiene, but according to studies on the moral development of children presented in 2010 at the University of Notre Dame, these original moms and dads raised well-adjusted, empathetic children.[1]

"They instinctively knew what was right for a child, and children thrived because of that," claims Darcia Narvaez, an associate professor of psychology at the University of Notre Dame, whose research on hunter-gatherer societies explored the psychological, anthropological, and biological conditions related to human development.

In certain ancient Semitic cultures of Mesopotamia, babies were named for the emotional response of the family upon the child's birth. Children modeled adults by playing with miniature weapons and household implements. Bonds between parents and children could be broken, as stated in Mesopotamian law: "If a son says to his father, 'You are not my father,' he can cut off his son's locks, make him a slave, and sell him for money. If a son says to his mother, 'You are not my mother,' she can cut off his locks, turn him out of town, or drive him away from home, deprive him of citizenship and inheritance, but his liberty he loses not. If a father says to his son, 'You are not my son,' the latter has to leave house and field, and he loses everything. If a mother says to her son, 'You are not my son,' he shall leave house and furniture."[2]

In classical Greece, babies who survived early infancy received toys during sacred festivals, and once they became adults, they dedicated their toys to various gods. Girls were kept at home until they married, but boys were encouraged to go to school and immerse themselves in the social world of their mentors.

During Roman times, the law and principle of *patria potestas* meant that the male head of household held absolute power over his children. He could discipline them as he wished, or even kill them or sell them into slavery. Valued children were given a *bulla*, or bag of magical charms worn around the neck to protect them from harm. Discipline could be harsh, but many Romans realized that the rod was counterproductive.

Imperial China valued its children highly. Parents debated philosophies of discipline and methods of character building, and many rulers encouraged a mix of harsh authority and gentle permissiveness.

Viking girls were educated in domestic arts, while boys typically learned farming. A community of adults raised these children together.

Skipping ahead to modern times (apologies to the amazing parents of the Coptic period in Egypt, the Persian Empire, China's Ming Dynasty, and the Dark Ages, just to name a few), we can understand today's parenting issues more thoroughly if we examine the changing conditions that precipitated most of the challenges we currently face. That will help us understand why parenting today is so hard and how we may ease that burden.

Life in America was great in the 1950s—if you were white, male, athletic, and popular. But other kids—nonwhite and not obviously athletic—had a much tougher time, and still do. While we have made many advances as a society regarding civil and human rights, making our country a better place for women, racial minorities, and the LGBT community, children have not necessarily reaped the benefits of this progress. Childhood anxiety, depression, suicides, and feelings of helplessness are on the rise, and these issues cut across race, economic class, and gender. It's wise not to take things for granted when it comes to the environment in which you are raising your children.

The Psychology of Children

It was barely one hundred years ago when scientific interest in parenting first began in America, with academic evaluation and recommendations for child rearing. Pediatrics, infant care, and child psychology became subjects of scientific interest only in the late 1800s. Up until then, health care for children was generally considered to fit within the confines of the church and the dominating trends of society.

The Industrial Revolution changed everything in America, with its great breakthroughs in technology, agriculture, and economic growth. But child labor became more rampant—and more harmful as well as more dangerous for children's well-being. In 1887 the American Pediatric Society was established to educate the general public on infant issues. They gradually started conducting baby examinations and expanded into childcare through adolescence. In 1897, the Parent Teacher Association was founded to advocate for children and their health and safety. In 1912, the US Children's Bureau was founded to provide information on infant care and maternal health matters.

From 1920 onward, American parents were privy to a host of information regarding their children's health. This science-based advice, however, was not always in the best interests of the children. Victorian behaviorist John Broadus Watson published his famous *Psychological Care of Infant and Child* in 1928, which presented his relatively rigid views on people and society.

"Treat them as though they were young adults," he wrote. "Dress them, bathe them with care and circumspection. Let your behavior always be objective and kindly and firm. Never hug and kiss them, never let them sit on your lap. Shake hands with them in the morning."[3]

Not exactly a ringing endorsement for affection. In fact, Watson advised parents to withhold that sort of love just in case it might spoil their children. He preferred that mothers and fathers reject their parental instincts, including any bonding on an emotional level, because he felt that any emotions, positive or negative, were a threat to order and rational behavior. By having parents act this way, Watson—and prominent others at the time who subscribed to his philosophy—felt that children would grow up with a sound work ethic and become more productive members of society.

Spock Talk

In his landmark 1946 book, *The Common Sense Book of Baby and Child Care*, Dr. Benjamin Spock, a disciple of the Freudian psychoanalyst view, encouraged mothers to trust rather than abandon their natural parenting instinct, a practice that John Broadus Watson had tried to eradicate. What distinguished Spock from others before him was his belief that if parents were going to better understand the behavior, needs, and personalities of their children, they would have to view the world from their children's perspective. Spock felt that being aware of and meeting a child's needs was crucial for the child's well-being and future development. Contrary to what has been said about Benjamin Spock, he did not suggest that parents abandon discipline. He favored methods of discipline that are age- and circumstance-appropriate, and not enforced merely for their own sake. He also preached about the importance of trying to understand what motivates a child's negative behavior and was a great supporter of affectionate parenting.

Children of the 1960s

Psychoanalyst John Bowlby offered the world his famous research on the early infant bonding process, including his theories of attachment, child grief, and separation. Yet another voice from the child-centered parenting domain was A. S. Neill, the Scottish educator and founder of the Summerhill School, a passionate advocate of a child's right to personal freedom. He said that "free children are not easily influenced; the absence of fear accounts for this phenomenon. Indeed, the absence of fear is the finest thing that can happen to a child."[4] He went on to add, "The function of the child is to live his own life, not the life that his anxious parents think he should live, nor a life according to the purpose of the educator who thinks he knows best."[5]

While both men, along with many other experts of their time, had a great influence on the progression of parenting philosophy in the United States, mixing the images of Victorian fathers and Freudian mothers, perhaps no one has had more influence than clinical and developmental psychologist Diana Baumrind, whose contributions to the field of child-rearing research are virtually unparalleled. She identifies the three most popular styles of parenting in white middle-class America in the 1960s as follows:

- **Authoritarian parenting:** A behaviorist parenting approach recommended by John Broadus Watson, utilizing high parental control and low parental responsiveness. This approach would be considered too strict and hard today.
- **Permissive parenting:** Inspired by the Freudian approach to children, urging low parental control and high parental responsiveness. Today, this approach would be considered too soft or permissive.
- **Authoritative parenting:** A combination of the two, featuring high parental control along with high parental responsiveness. This approach is now considered to be just the right balance of authoritarian and permissive parenting.

This is how Diana Baumrind describes the role of the mother:

> She encourages verbal give and take, and shares with the child the reasoning behind her policy. She values both expressive and instrumental attributes, both autonomous self-will and disciplined conformity. Therefore, she exerts firm control at points of parent-child divergence, but does not hem the child in with restrictions. She recognizes her own special rights as an adult, but also the child's individual interests and special ways. The authoritative parent affirms the child's present qualities, but also sets standards for future conduct. She uses reason as well as power to achieve her objectives. She does not base her decisions on group consensus or the individual child's desires; but also does not regard herself as infallible or divinely inspired.[6]

The Changing Paradigm of Parenting

What worked in previous generations doesn't necessarily hold up so well with today's crop of parents. What used to be nonnegotiable between parents and children, such as bedtime, attire, and cleaning your plate at the dinner table, is now open for discussion in many households. Quite often, it's much more tempting (and easier) for parents to just give in, give up, or go along with their child's wishes, as if they were not the parents, or don't want to continue to reinforce traditional ideas and values. Nowadays, parents are more willing to blame someone else for whatever shortcomings or issues they perceive their children to be facing, even when they are self-inflicted or precipitated by the parent and/or child.

Of course, many people claim a multitude of fundamental reasons for why parenting today is so hard. From the parents, educators, and professional family experts to whom we have spoken, here is a short list of what they report:

1. Parents' careers are more complicated or demanding.
2. Times are more dangerous.
3. Families don't live near each other, compromising the input and help from an extended family.
4. Parents want their child to be seen as "perfect."
5. Parents need full access all the time to everyone in their child's school.
6. Everyone is expected to go to college, and to the "right" college.
7. Parents expect their children to do something significant after college.
8. Smaller family size creates more pressure on their child to "make it" in the world.
9. Parents are afraid that their kids won't be successful by their definition.
10. Kids today are less responsible and have little sense of boundaries.
11. There is a much higher number of single parents and children of divorce.

This list is surely incomplete, but collectively it still demonstrates a relatively narrow view of why parenting in today's world is so hard. Let's see if any of these reasons really stand up upon closer inspection:

1. Parents' careers are not necessarily more complicated, but in our current economy, they may be more demanding, especially when it comes to overtime.

2. Times seem more dangerous in some parts of America because of the proliferation of guns, but, generally speaking, the crime rate has gone down.

3. Families don't live near each other. As our society becomes more mobile, the extended family unit has disintegrated and childcare has become less of an "inside job," with fewer family relatives participating. Although many people live near each other in big cities, it seems like fewer and fewer people get to know each other, much less trust each other to help look after their children.

4. Parents want their child to be seen as "perfect," certainly by others. This is nothing new, but it's still a factor, especially among those parents who feel as if they can buy, hire, or coach perfection.

5. Parents need full access all the time to everyone in their child's school. First of all, unfettered access would be a nightmare for teachers and administrators, and it would do little good for the students. Parents who feel this way might benefit from seeking a new hobby, therapy, or vice in place of their children.

6. Everyone is expected to go to college, and to the "right" college, too, not just any old school. The pressure on families to have their kids attend college has grown exponentially, and for good reason. In today's workforce, a college degree is essentially equivalent to what a high school diploma was two generations ago. On top of that, there is a greater push than ever among upwardly mobile parents to get their kids into "elite" colleges and universities. This is causing an enormous upheaval throughout America's educational system and an ever-growing cottage industry of tutors, consultants, and

literature on the subject of getting your child into "the right school."

7. Parents expect their children to do something valuable and productive after college. The race is on to get the best jobs after school. Unfortunately, the unemployment numbers for college graduates seem to be rising.

8. Smaller families put more pressure on their child to "make it" in the world. Logically, parents tend to focus more on only children, and because today's families are generally smaller, this is causing a general increase in overparenting.

9. Parents are afraid that their kids won't be successful. This fear can be traced back to the Depression era and Post-Depression, when parents were afraid that their children might suffer the same setbacks they did as children.

10. Kids today feel less responsible and have little sense of boundaries. This may apply to children who have been spoiled and feel a certain sense of entitlement, but it is not always the case and certainly occurs less often inside intact, well-grounded households.

11. There are more single parents and more divorced families, but that does not mean that parents can't learn to co-parent and work things out for the benefit of the children.

Honestly, a number of the reasons for overparenting stated by those we surveyed made some sense, and may suggest reasonable, understandable challenges; however, each of them is controllable and need not become an obstacle to healthy parenting.

Who's Minding the Store?

The late Suzanne Bianchi, a social scientist who analyzed how American families have changed during the late twentieth century, found that working mothers of the 1990s spent as much time (an average of twelve hours) with their children as—or more than—stay-at-home mothers of the 1960s.[7] This challenges the perception most of us have developed that today's working women may be short-changing their children of what they purportedly need to ensure proper nourishment. In fact, Bianchi discovered that working mothers today spend the same amount of time (an average of twelve hours) with their children as their counterparts during the 1960s.

So how can mothers (and fathers) effectively parent their children if they are spending more and more time away from home—working? Common sense would have us believe that less time at home means something negative for children. However, the math doesn't always work out that way. In many cases, time is simply spent differently. Parents sleep less, delegate housework, eat out less, cut back on TV time and "date nights," work a certain amount of hours from a home office, and in households with small children they occasionally bring their kids to work. It's a matter of shifting gears and managing time and space effectively. It sure sounds easy enough. We wonder why more parents aren't following this path.

We can argue quite confidently that over the past fifteen to twenty years these parental tendencies have shifted and, in many cases, not necessarily for the better. Many, if not most, parents work more than thirty hours per week; working forty, fifty, and even sixty hours is not uncommon for parents in demanding professions. Children may be compromised when both of their parents are gone at work for a good portion of their children's waking hours.

Some parents actively seek promotions, which will mean increased time away from their families but more money in the bank, along with the possibility of affording private school and a private university for their kids.

Raising a Global Child in Today's Society

The responsibility of raising our children does not fall on the shoulders of parents alone. Between home, school, television, the Internet, and Madison Avenue, your child is bombarded on a daily basis by passive and active external forces, some rather aggressive and invasive. As a parent, you're the quarterback of a team. In the beginning, you control how your children eat, what they wear, and with whom and where they hang out. Slowly but surely, that changes as they begin attending school, unless, of course, you live in the woods, free of electronic devices. By the time your child becomes a teenager, you may control the purse strings and the curfew but not much else.

Mission impossible? Welcome to raising a global child in today's society. It *is* hard, but it's all a matter of letting go—in a positive sense. Your children can certainly learn from you; you are probably the first presenter of a moral code in life and their primary role model, but you are far from the only one! The sooner you realize that fact about you and your children, the better off all of you will be. This reality is not much different than it has always been, but there are significantly more external inputs now than ever before.

This means that beginning with your babysitter or nanny, you rapidly cease to be the only adult or outside influence in your child's life. How, then, can you manage what your child digests, much less his or her evolving emancipation? What about the risk factors that accompany your child's increased freedom? Are you willing to accept that as your children age and develop, life becomes more risky and you control less and less of it?

Those are tough pills to swallow. Without any formal education in parenting, how are we supposed to know how to do it? Shall we simply copy and, in some cases, emulate what our parents did—for better or for worse? We can read one or two of the plethora of books available, and that can be quite helpful, but, overall, we must choose what type of parent we want to be, based on our own personalities, strengths, and weaknesses and our understanding of our environment and our children.

The Big Three Parenting Styles

Just as we have presented a host of parenting archetypes and styles, a deeper evaluation of their combined consequences may be merited. Diane Baumrind has coupled some of these tendencies in ways that clearly reveal the pitfalls of overparenting:

- **Authoritarian Parenting:** This is generally considered to be an oppressive parenting style that may have unfortunate long-term consequences for children, producing low self-esteem and poor social skills.

- **Authoritarian Beliefs and Values:** Patriarchy, Victorian ideals, behaviorism, insensitivity and intolerance, hierarchy, authority, submissiveness, harshness, predictability, conservatism, no parent-child discussions, a black-and-white world view, rigidity, aggressiveness, inhibiting psychological control, suppression of emotions, threats.

- **Permissive Parenting:** This style has been noted for producing children with good social skills and high self-esteem but mediocre academic performance. Therefore, this parenting style is also seen as less successful because, in general, academic performance is considered to be a goal.

- **Permissive Beliefs and Values:** Freudianism, manipulative control, bribes, individual autonomy and personal freedom, high creativity, non-restrictiveness, role equality, non-punitive techniques, harmony-orientated environment, free development, flat hierarchy, self-regulation.

- **Authoritative Parenting:** This is considered to be the most successful of the three parenting styles in terms of producing happy, independent children who do well in school.

- **Authoritative Beliefs and Values:** Social responsibility, shaping and reinforcement, cooperation, rational control, relative freedom of choice.

- **Shared Authoritarian and Authoritative Beliefs and Values:** High behavior control, disciplined conformity, demands and chores, rules and order, obedience, punishments.

- **Shared Authoritative and Permissive Beliefs and Values:** High responsiveness, give-and-take discussions, self-assertiveness, warmth, independent thinking, meeting needs, encouragement.[8]

Mindful Parenting

Which parenting style or combination of styles do you prefer? Which might work best for you? The only way to determine that is to be in the moment as much as possible, and that means finding a balance between establishing a consistent parenting style and living life as it happens, one minute, one hour, and one day at a time. If you can do that, if you can be aware of your feelings as they ebb and flow—and change—parenting won't feel so hard, and communication with your children will get easier and produce better results.

Following someone else's rules will only get you so far. You must get in touch with yourself as a parent, much like you had to do when you first moved away from your parents' home and, inspired by your upbringing, established your own identity and presence in the world. Listening to yourself is a start, after which you must follow your intuition and learn as you grow. Sometimes, in order to feel secure, your child will need you to be predictable and set well-established boundaries, while at other times he or she may need freedom and the chance to take risks and possibly even fail! That's right. Sometimes, the best thing you can do is get out of the way and let your kid make his or her own choices, even if you can see that the child may not get it right. That may be your biggest challenge and what many parents are unconsciously referring to when they say that parenting is hard, or "it will hurt me more than it hurts you." Letting go and allowing your children to make their own choices and fail—while you watch— is a big challenge. From your perspective, it means paying attention, opening your heart, negotiating, and making decisions. Then, it will require yielding, one of the hardest thing for any parent to do sincerely and successfully.

"When we took our ninth-grade daughter to a boarding school and were about to say goodbye," reports Tabitha, a mother of two from Tampa, Florida, "I couldn't help noticing how small she appeared, especially with all the upperclassmen running around the campus. She wanted to be there, but I was nearly trembling, imagining how she would cope with so much newness in her young life. Just as we were about to go, I ran to the car to make sure we hadn't forgotten anything. I think I was trying to escape the moment of saying goodbye. As I was about to leave, my older son gave me some great advice: 'Mom, whatever you feel like telling my sister right now—don't. No words of wisdom before you drive away, leaving her in tears. She won't cry. She's totally fine. Let's just say goodbye and go.' So that's what we did, and we are all better for it."

Your Child's School as Co-Parent

An effective parent must learn to yield. Recognizing that your time parenting your children is limited and that it is augmented by a variety of other individuals and institutions is an important part of being able to let go. This does not occur only at home. Parental yielding goes far beyond your efforts at home. On an average weekday, your elementary- to high-school-age children spend approximately seven hours at their respective schools, and up to three more hours if they participate in afterschool activities, such as pottery class, drama, homework help, or athletics. Their school plays a significant role in helping you bring up your children. Therefore, your relationship with that school can influence your child's overall experience.

As a parent, you must learn to navigate your way through an ever-changing educational system influenced by federal, state, and local mandates that can affect everything from a school's social culture to its testing philosophy and practice. Your involvement is up to you. Certainly, it's good to know what's going on, but becoming too present is not advisable. It's your child's school. When a teacher takes attendance, it is your child's name that is called out, and unless a problem develops, your child's teacher does not need to know you very well.

Trust: that's what it's all about. It doesn't matter whether you are sending your child to a public or private school; you must take a leap of faith and trust the school to do what it theoretically knows how to do: educate your child. Sure, pay attention and keep up with the daily, weekly, or monthly goings on, but, as a rule, it's best to not interfere with your child's school experience, unless, of course, he or she is obviously struggling with an academic, social, or physical issue.

Most French children wave goodbye to their parents at age two or three when they enter France's educational machine and embark on a path intended to make them into miniature adults. This is true in many countries, especially where both parents traditionally hold jobs and need daycare for their children at a very young age.

So, do schools really take care of your children? Can they be consistent with your parenting style at home? It seems that schools are not as strict as they used to be. We rarely see children walking around with bruised knuckles and sore backsides as a result of corporal punishment. That's a good thing, of course, but an increase in parental involvement in their children's school activities often is a result of a lack of respect, prestige, and recognition for teachers, which in turn leads to a decline in teachers' authority over children at school. When we speak of our children displaying bad behavior, who is responsible, and where and how can it be remedied? Some parents drop off their kids at school and expect the teachers to take care of everything—teaching values, good behavior, how to dress, what to eat, and so on—from soup to nuts, and then reinforce that stuff as well!

"I pay the school all this money, so they ought to raise my kid," says Bill, an oil executive in Dallas, Texas, who sends his son to a local private school. Does Bill have unreasonable expectations and a misguided sense of entitlement? Probably, but he's not the only one—by far—and it's not just private school parents who take this stance. Plenty of PTA folks in public schools are guilty of the same behavior, in effect, abdicating their responsibility, *under*parenting their children, and then wanting to blame someone beside themselves if they don't like how their children turned out.

Parent-teacher conferences may not happen often enough for some parents, but in most schools teachers encourage parents to email them with any concerns. Thank goodness for email. It keeps overly anxious parents at bay and from randomly barging into the classroom, at least to a point. Beyond that communication, some schools provide parents with the option of using specialized recordkeeping software to access the schools' websites and monitor their children's grades and class attendance. Parents can also check on what their kids are eating by monitoring their children's lunch menu through special websites. These services go a long way toward keeping you informed, and then helping you determine when to advocate for your child and when to yield.

These days, though, despite having all this information available, parents have become increasingly involved in activities and decisions that were previously under the teachers' absolute discretion and control. Parental involvement also extends to school governance and decisions pertaining to curricular and extracurricular activities. Surely you've seen more than your fair share of parents intervening on their children's behalf to ensure that they get their first choice in selecting their child's teacher for the next year, or which extracurricular activities their child can participate in. In some cases, parents who go too far could be accused of bullying their children's school.

But it doesn't have to be this way. What can schools do to combat overparenting? Even more important, what can you do to ensure that you aren't already or won't become one of these parents? How can you empower yourself to establish boundaries between you and your child's school, much like you try to teach your child to do? If you think you have it rough, imagine what a typical school goes through, trying to educate masses of children, while doing its best to satisfy hundreds, if not thousands, of demanding parents, who are often not as knowledgeable as they think.

Ban Those Balls!

Going overboard in the pursuit of protecting our children is not limited to parental behavior. With the omnipresent fear of litigation, schools can be equally guilty of "overprotecting the children," as exhibited recently by school officials at Weber Middle School in Port Washington, New York. It seems that some students were getting hurt during recess, and according to school superintendent Kathleen Maloney, "some of these injuries can unintentionally become very serious, so we want to make sure our children have fun, but are also protected."[9]

As a result, footballs, baseballs, lacrosse balls, and any other balls that could possibly hurt someone are banned on school grounds. Physical tag games are also verboten, as are unsupervised cartwheels. It's not clear if spontaneous jumping for joy will continue to be allowed, but if these measures are any indication, that too may also soon be banned, and it won't be because some kids are simply awkward.

While it's clear that helmets and pads can help prevent injuries, we haven't been able to find many statistics to support the dangers of unsupervised cartwheels. In fact, it's hard to understand why this has even happened, and why other school districts are apparently considering following suit. Playground injuries are as old as playgrounds, and most playgrounds these days, with their rubberized flooring, are infinitely safer than they used to be. So, is this concern for safety going too far? If a child breaks his leg playing kickball, do you cancel all kickball games for the foreseeable future and ban kickballs altogether? If a kid falls off a jungle gym in a playground and cracks his elbow, do you immediately have the jungle gyms removed, or only allow a child on one if there is an adult monitor at his or her side? Or, to go even further, do you simply close all playgrounds? At Weber Middle School, that's what the administration has effectively done. Perhaps because Port Washington, like any other town, has its share of car accidents, it won't be long before it will be banning cars.

Childhood is fraught with danger. But are Nerf balls really the answer for everything?

"Hey, Tommy, go out for a pass!" says Dave.

"OK, sure, Dave, here I go!" Tommy replies.

Tommy, all four-foot-three of him, goes racing across the playground, zigzagging his way through the other children, who are peacefully playing kickball with a balloon.

"I'm throwing you this Nerf football, Tommy," yells Dave to his friend. "Keep running and look, come on, look for the ball, it's coming! Hey, Tommy! Watch out! Be careful; you're going to run into the fence!"

Which is exactly what Tommy does, after he bangs into his teacher and crashes into the fence, just as the Nerf ball safely bonks him on the head.

This sounds like a scene straight out of *The Nerf Ball From Hell*, just another case of institutionalized over-adulting. Let kids be kids! Good manners and human decency are one thing, but too much political correctness is another. By enacting these rules, the school district in Port Washington has legally wussified an entire town.

Think how far some parents may take the situation:

"I'm very upset," says Carmine, an imaginary mother of three from Port Washington. "My son was playing baseball the other day at school, and they were using a tomato instead of a ball. Anyway, he's up at bat, and the pitcher hits him in the eye with the tomato!

At first, he's not hurt, but then his eye swells up and he has to go to the emergency room. It turns out he has lycopene poisoning. If the school would have been using a baseball like kids have been doing for the past one hundred years, my son could have just gotten a plain old concussion instead of lycopene poisoning! I mean, he could have died from that!"

We are not advocating negligence or carelessness. We also recommend that children wear batting helmets, even when using vegetables or fruits to replace actual baseballs. However, we do encourage a healthy dose of reality, risk, acceptance, and common sense.

Whose Education Is This, Anyway?

Some parents become too involved in their children's educational experience. They push administrations to assign their children to the "best" teacher in a particular grade, berate coaches for not playing their children enough on an athletic team, or intervene when it comes time for casting the school play. They may even uproot their family and move to a new part of town with what is perceived to be a better school, in spite of the children's wish to remain in a neighborhood that they consider to be home. This is often accompanied by a succession of tutors and private coaches, beginning at an early age and continuing all the way through high school.

Some kids are naturally more gifted athletically than others, just as some are more academically adroit. Children develop at different speeds, so a child who physically develops very rapidly may be slower to catch up intellectually. This process, which reflects the neurological system's maturation, is frequently more obvious with boys than with girls. In spite of that, some parents expect—and push for—their children to excel at everything, and all at the same time! Interestingly, this is particularly true for parents who were not stars growing up but wished they were and now hope that they can push their children into accomplishing what they couldn't.

This may mean hiring a private baseball coach for a six-year-old by a father who never played or was a marginal junior high school player. While he knows nothing about coaching, this parent will maneuver his way into becoming the Little League coach, not because he particularly wants to volunteer, but so that his son can be the team's starting pitcher.

Behavior like this can happen on a larger scale, too. In a suburban Pennsylvania town a few years ago, several parents hired two semipro ball players to coach their children's team, whereas all the other teams in the league used local college kids, most of whom had played on the same field when they were growing up. The team with the fancy coaches did not win many more games, but it created a lot of animosity with the other parents, and a sense of unfairness to the children on the other teams. Despite the use of semipro coaches, no one from that team, or, in fact, any of the other teams, ever made it to the major leagues, and it is unlikely that anyone will. But all it took to create this situation was a few parents who were aging, frustrated jocks and were willing to do anything to give their kids a leg up on the competition.

Pursuing a better education or athletic advantage for children—at any cost—can be harmful to the very children parents are trying so hard to support. Parents must allow their children to learn the lay of the land—that not everyone can be the star of the play or the team, and that failure can be as valuable a lesson, if not more so, than success. Children already know who is good and bad at different things, be it in sports, academics, or school, and sometimes not intervening allows them to appreciate the gifts that others have, and in turn to value their own talents, which is a much more important life lesson. While it may hurt at the time, most children figure out that, as Mick and Keith once told us, "you can't always get what you want" all of the time.

Managing Expectations

"My kid is only a tree in the first-grade play," Ray said, feeling as if his whole world was being cut out from underneath him. "I need to talk to somebody to get him a better part."

Really? The insanity has begun! Ray is making things difficult for his child, and his kid is only in first grade! This has trouble written all over it. We can safely bet that Ray loves his kid and wants the best for him, but why is he already freaking out because his son will be playing a tree in the school play? Maybe it's a story about trees, and he's the star tree who sings and dances! Who knows? Maybe he *is* just playing a glorified piece of furniture. So what? Are the other children performing soliloquies at his expense? No wonder parenting is so hard. Ray is making it impossibly difficult because of his unrealistic expectations. He's obsessing about his son's success for absolutely no reason.

How do we get parents like Ray to manage their expectations for their kids? How do we get parents to manage their own expectations? Can we just say to these parents, "Your kid is not a genius! There's only one Einstein. Not every child is meant to go to Harvard; not every kid is meant to play major-league baseball. Get over it; average is beautiful. Appreciate the abilities that he or she has, not the ones you want him to have." Can we actually say that? When it comes to our own children, can we hear it and accept it? Let's hope so. Let's hope that we can accept, appreciate, and honor the gifts that each of our children possesses, even if they are not the ones that we thought he or she should have.

It would be wise to learn from our ancient predecessors. Our forefathers and mothers, the hunters and gatherers, nurtured their offspring with kindness and hours of unstructured free play. In fact, children were raised in a village atmosphere, with multiple adult caretakers. That guaranteed a certain level of physical affection and comfort, which pediatricians agree is crucial during a child's developing years.

Sounds like common sense, but not everyone gets it. In fact, many parents need to be reminded—and in some cases, taught—how to love their children, by simply being there for them and providing a loving, caring environment.

There is no "I" in "Team"—or "Parent." So, let us be clear as parents that our children's lives are *their* lives and not ours. We already have our own, and by the grace of God we are simply here to enjoy the privilege of watching (and sometimes helping) these human beings discover themselves, sometimes right in front of our eyes. Enjoy it. Love and appreciate the journey. It doesn't have to be as hard as you make it out to be.

Overparenting or Just Plain Dumb?

In this game, you will read examples of parental behavior and decide whether the mom or dad in the story is overparenting (OP) or just plain dumb (JPD). What do you win? Peace of mind, confidence, and the knowledge that you're not screwing up your kids too badly.

(Please note: These questions are rhetorical and do not suggest actual answers.)

1. A parent wrote her child's paper, and the child received a grade of C. The parent was upset, and, as it turns out, she had consulted with an out-of-state professor to get his ideas for the paper. It's unknown whether the professor was also given a C or was asked for a refund because his work did not get the desired result.

Is this an example of overparenting (OP) or just plain dumb (JPD)?

2. A high school student was having trouble in school and skipped some classes, but as a cheerleader she was intent on showing up at the homecoming game. However, she missed school for a second day, saying that she had to go to the Department of Public Safety for her driver's license. The school called home to say that because of the absences, no matter what the reason, she couldn't cheer at the weekend game. Her mother pleaded her daughter's case, lying about her daughter's whereabouts on the day she missed school. But because her daughter had been caught on video getting her nails done in a salon during school hours, the mother's cover-up backfired. She got mad at the school for not understanding that as a cheerleader her daughter needed her nails to look perfect for the game.

Is this an example of overparenting (OP) or just plain dumb (JPD)?

3. A seventeen-year-old boy has grown up quite smothered and spoiled. He goes on a community service school project to Kenya, where his school and his parents hope that he will learn a few life lessons. At the last minute, however, the boy's parents go with him, which in essence undoes the potential for having a positive effect on the child.

Is this an example of overparenting (OP) or just plain dumb (JPD)?

4. A mother with a heavyset daughter wants her school and a counselor to put the kid on a diet and help her pick out her clothes, rather than the mom being the one to tell her daughter that she is overweight, and doing these activities with her.

Is this an example of overparenting (OP) or just plain dumb (JPD)?

5. John is a six-foot-two-inch, 210-pound high school senior. One day, with his class scheduled to leave in the morning on a field trip, he goes to school without his lunch. That morning, both his parents noticed that John had forgotten his lunch, so each of them drives to the school with an alternative meal. Neither parent could imagine

John's missing lunch that day, even though the school had already told the parents that it would be providing pizza on the bus. John's father drops off a lunch for his son and heads back to work. John's mother breaks down in the school office.

"I'm really sorry," she says, "but besides taking care of my husband and kids, I don't have much of a life."

Is this an example of overparenting (OP) or just plain dumb (JPD)?
6. At one particular private school, student grades are posted online every day. When parents check in, some of them call and/or text their kids during the school day to tell them their grades, and, if it applies, they even will ask them what they did to mess up. Others contact the school directly, even before their children know what is going on, to challenge the grades and demand changes.

Is this an example of overparenting (OP) or just plain dumb (JPD)?
7. Valerie is in fifth grade, and she isn't doing very well in school, which upsets her mother, who demands a meeting with all of Valerie's teachers. She wants them all to sign a contract, promising that her daughter will get good enough grades to be admitted into a prestigious middle school.

Is this an example of overparenting (OP) or just plain dumb (JPD)?
8. Scott has been removed from his school play because of his bad attendance record and poor grades. His parents write a letter to the editor of the local newspaper, blaming it all on the school and claiming that being in the play is the only thing their child likes or is good at, and if the school deprives him of that, they will be doing irreparable harm to his future.

Is this an example of overparenting (OP) or just plain dumb (JPD)?
9. Candice let her nine-year-old son ride the New York City subway alone. This caused an uproar among local parents and was even picked up by international media. When Candice appeared on a national TV

program to discuss her decision to let her son ride the subway alone, the host asked the viewers at home whether Valerie was "an enlightened mom or a really bad one."[10]

Is the media reaction an example of overparenting (OP) or just plain dumb (JPD)?

10. At a recent gathering of kindergarten parents at a small school, the teacher pointed out one child's painting among others hanging on the walls of an exhibit displaying all the children's artwork.

"He's a gifted artist," the teacher announced to everyone.

The "gifted" child's father raced home and told his son what happened. He then proceeded to find art tutors for his son, promising him that they would help him draw even better. His son looked at him like he was an alien.

"Dad, I just wanna draw stuff, OK?"

Is this an example of overparenting (OP) or just plain dumb (JPD)?

The Ethical Road Is Forked

Whether we refer to certain parental behavior as overparenting or just plain dumb, the choices that parents make are often rooted in the moral code that they opt to adopt. Most of us learn basic concepts of right and wrong when we are young children, taught by our parents, in fact, and later embellished by relatives, teachers, coaches, and mentors. These lessons form the foundation of our value systems, as tried and true for us as the Ten Commandments. For many parents, though, these principles, such as "do unto others as you would have done to you," fall by the wayside, often as early as when it's time to find a spot in a preferred preschool program. At that point, some parents (unbeknownst to their children, so it's OK in their minds) go to great lengths to gain their children's admittance. In New York City, parents have been known to grease the palms of admissions directors for a spot in a select school, much like prospective tenants have been doing with building superintendents for years to secure an apartment over other candidates. "Do whatever it takes" is the familiar refrain in those circumstances, but who are we convincing when we tell ourselves that as parents? Does the end really justify the means? What kind of hypocrisy are we setting ourselves up for when it comes to raising our kids?

"Do what I say, not what I do." Really? Has parenting become so hard these days that we have to lie and cheat to help our kids get ahead? Is the ethical road as forked as it appears? Each of us must answer that question as we navigate our way through this complicated thing called parenting.

CHAPTER 3: HOW DOES OVERPARENTING HAPPEN?

In the United States, overparenting seems to have started with the Baby Boomer generation, when folks grew up in a world of increasing access to education, job security, wealth, and technology. But in the span of a few decades, the Baby Boomers' offspring have morphed into a society built on vanity, consumerism, an acceptance of excess, reduced attention spans, and a sense that there are shortcuts to almost everything. We were told that we could be anybody and do anything.

"Just do it."

"Be all that you can be."

"Think outside the box."

The encouragement from Madison Avenue is quite seductive and continues to influence one generation after the next.

"Have it your way."

"The power to be your best."

"Unleash the beast."

"Life's a sport. Drink it up."

"The best never rest."

These messages seem to be speaking to each and every one of us, hitting our empathy bones and anointing us with the capability to rule the world, or at least our local universe, or at least our child's school, or, at the very least, our own home.

"Impossible is nothing."

"Success. It's a mind game."

"Because you're worth it."

With all these encouraging words, it's no wonder that some parents simply feel entitled, especially if their world is expanding materialistically and they anoint themselves as unofficial masters of the universe, believing that their children are entitled to the same benefits, luxuries, and preferential treatment that they are experiencing.

On the other hand, many parents are seeing their world shrink, as jobs go overseas, education becomes more difficult to obtain, and families get smaller. Parents threatened by economic woes are afraid that their kids may not be successful. Understandably, they will do anything to provide their children with a chance to enhance their position in life and succeed.

Defining Success

Is it a success when parents hire a team of tutors for their child to whip her into shape academically so that she will achieve test scores beyond her natural capacity, opening the door to get her into a college that is too big of a reach, where she will not succeed on her own? For a child who has had everything managed for her all through childhood, how will she automatically know how to manage her own time, let alone keep up with the academic demands of a high-quality university, without that team of tutors holding her hand and guiding her every step of the way? Is it any wonder that in this era, more than 50 percent of all college students require at least five years to graduate?

According to a high school college counselor we spoke to in the fall of 2014, "I have parents bringing in completed college applications that they filled out for their child—including the essays! In this society fueled by wealth and status, the father's job is to make a lot of money so that the family can continue to live in the right neighborhood and go to the right school, while the mother's job is to make the children successful. If the mother doesn't succeed with her kid, meaning get him or her into an elite college, then the mother is considered a failure. In these social circles, we have seen marriages deteriorate, where the father may even divorce the mother because she did not do her job well when the child does not meet his expectations. We have also seen situations where a father loses his job, meaning that they can no longer live in the right part of town and their child can no longer attend an exclusive school, and the father, unable to bear what he perceives to be an embarrassing change in circumstances, commits suicide. In other instances, even when something so drastic does not occur, it can cause complete family breakdowns."

Insecure parents are rolling their problems onto their children. Perhaps these parents grew up without positive parental role models, because it's clear that they don't know how to be appropriate role models for their children. Why have parents become so desperate to have their kids attend prestigious colleges that they will go to almost any length to make that happen, beginning when the children are so young that they have not yet learned to read?

The competition to get into college is essentially out of control at this point. With more and more applicants each year to colleges and universities, these schools can be more selective than ever. Many of today's parents are so obsessed with paving a path for their children's automatic success that they do not give their kids even a remote, selective chance to fail. This is really too bad, because it's especially easy to fix many of the failures and use them as a learning experience for our children. If parents would occasionally do this, we might see them redefining success—for themselves and, even better, for their overparented kids. It is important to recognize that when children are little, their mistakes and failures are small and relatively easy to correct. When they get older, and their mistakes and failures often become bigger, the efforts to correct them also become more difficult.

One of the great comforts of parenting is that we don't always have to focus on ourselves and our own shortcomings. Instead, we can become very busy taking care of our kids in the hopes that they will make up for our own disappointments! Being responsible feels so good—at first—but then it can quickly become something else, like an obsession. But why? Why do parents become so obsessed with their kids? What drives parents to behave like that?

"This is our only child. We've got to get it right."

We've heard this refrain a million times. Let's see where it was born.

In the Beginning

Your first child has just been born. Your hopes and dreams are booming, like the most optimistic fireworks display on the Fourth of July. You bring your baby home, swaddled in a safety net of abundant love. You want the best for him, no matter what. Everything should be perfectly safe and smooth with no bumps or bruises—none.

When your parents and in-laws arrive, they coo and cuddle and admire your prodigious ability to procreate. Everyone toasts to the newborn's future, to his or her future acceptance at Harvard, to finding the right spouse and a top career, with a large house full of perfect children and a life of success and happiness. Your kid is barely forty-eight hours old, and you're already planning his entire life!

For some anxious parents, this marks the first stage of overparenting. This is especially true for a parent raising his or her first child. Each time the baby burps, the parent may flinch and consider running to the emergency room. But by the time that same parent has a second or third child, it's usually quite a different story. Burping, falling, and crying—the usual range of daily angst and agitation—often become quite unremarkable for a parent of multiple children.

"Since my son was born a few years ago," says Paul, an architect in Charlotte, North Carolina, "all the crazy technology we're surrounded with has only given me more stuff to obsess about. For example, I recently noticed a recall alert for our jogging stroller on my Facebook page, describing how the product label could be removed, becoming a potential object for a baby to choke on. They said that no baby had actually choked yet, but I certainly didn't want my son to be the first. It seems like from the day he was born, I have been on involuntary lookout for anything that could possibly go wrong or harm him in any way, big or small. I've investigated every alarm system for his room in our house and researched pollution detectors and car seats till I can't keep my eyes open at the computer. Now, I read every warning on every label of every object I purchase. My son is six months old. I can't imagine how crazy I will become by the time he's walking."

Caution: Fragile Contents Inside

Are your kids really as fragile as you think they are? For some people, overparenting begins at birth, when parents begin overprotecting their children with an unnecessary amount of swaddling. This continues with enlisting baby coaches, enrolling in pre-toddler tutoring programs, and cajoling pediatricians to prescribe needless antibiotics.

Your expectations may be as fragile as your child's two-year-old little body. What happens when he or she doesn't meet your expectations, which will undoubtedly happen sooner or later? How do you react when one of your children doesn't get a leg up on the competition?

The answers to these questions may be found in how you were raised by your parents. Many of us, despite how well our parents may have done in bringing us up, still feel a need to do better. For those whose childhood memories remain full of the fallout from a divorce, preoccupied parents, countless hours of solitary activity in front of the television, and a freezer full of TV dinners, it's no wonder that they are determined—if not obsessed—with winning a Parent of the Year award *every* year and for every child. They feel a need to make up for what they missed, thought they missed, or consider to have been a less than optimal childhood. But was that childhood really so awful? Previous generations enjoyed freedoms that don't come easily in contemporary society. Walking to school alone, with time to reflect or just happily space out, seems like a bygone luxury for many kids today. Imagine your child taking her time to stroll home after school, unattended, and then spending hours in the backyard with nothing special to do and no one checking every fifteen minutes to make sure that she's properly stimulated and fed.

We are not advising that you abandon your children and let them fend for themselves. But a parent can be present without being intrusive. It's a dance that we all should pay attention to and do our best to master. It requires observation, watching, listening, and developing a feel for when we should engage and when we should yield to the ebb and flow of a developing individual. When in doubt, ask. Children of all ages have a fairly keen sense of when they want company, when they want help, and when they are just fine being alone.

Regardless of whether you are the child of a divorce or not, it's no surprise that you feel committed to making your child's life as perfect as possible. Many of you probably made a vow with yourself that if you ever had kids, you would never argue with your spouse in front of your children, let alone get divorced. Your home would be stable and loving, a creative and nourishing place for children to grow up and flourish in. Whatever shortcomings your parents may have had, you would not only erase them; you would obliterate them in a nonstop clinic in how to be an *amazing* parent, also known as Super Mom or Super Dad, shield optional.

Aspirations like these are fine, but the consequences of being overzealous should be somewhat obvious by now. We can't become better parents by controlling our kids' childhoods. We must be willing to let them play in the backyard without our micromanagement and devoted attention, leaving them the opportunity to discover their own shortcomings, creativity, hungers, and strengths. You can begin to practice this hands-on/hands-off approach at an early age, giving your children the gift of independence.

Testing! Testing! Testing!

When parents start testing their children as early as possible, without a clear-cut medical reason and without a physician's referral, who really benefits? The testing centers certainly do, but who else? Depending on the results of the tests, which can so often be skewed, particularly by a testing facility that also provides follow-up training or therapy, the information the tests reveal can be particularly suspect when we're talking about a child who may barely be speaking, and the parent's reaction to the test results can range from great satisfaction to abject panic.

"If my child's test results are off the charts," says Brian, an economics professor at a Southern university, "should I be bringing in specialized tutors right away to make sure he realizes his apparently huge potential?"

"What if my child doesn't test well?" asks Claudia, a computer software executive from the Northeast. "Should I hire tutors to help her correct her deficits?"

Once they submit their kids to testing, Brian and Claudia are stuck with their scores and with a diagnosis that the child may be given. As parents they are cursed, because they are attaching great meaning to the numbers and looking to take immediate action, whether it's to get the most out of their little Einstein or to "correct" their "deficit-laden" child.

Short of avoiding the whole testing merry-go-round, how can parents navigate through the pressures of getting their children into the best preschools, which is seen as the ticket to the best elementary schools, middle schools, colleges, and ultimately graduate schools? No one can question a parent who wants the best for his or her child, but at what expense? What's reasonable when it comes to testing? At what age should the testing start? And what should parents do when their child's initial tests don't meet their hopes and expectations? Maybe parents should be tested, too, so that we can be sure that their children will be protected as they grow up, in spite of their parents' overzealous behavior. In the case of a two- to five-year-old, the more accurate testing would be of the parents, their IQ, and their ability to function in the world, rather than testing the children. Imagine if gynecologists were charged with testing each pregnant woman (and partner, when available) who was in the process of becoming a parent? The following parental aptitude test (PAT) may reveal crucial areas in which prospective parents need help, and why not provide that assistance before it's too late?

Parental Aptitude Test

(answers on page 194)

1. Successful parenting means:
   A. Your children attend Ivy League schools and become doctors or lawyers.
   B. Your children take care of you when you get old.
   C. Your children enjoy growing up and feel good about themselves.

    D. Your children become so independent that they move out by age thirteen.

2. Children should be seen, heard, or tested.
    A. Seen.
    B. Heard.
    C. Tested.
    D. All of the above.

3. If your child breastfeeds, it means that he will:
    A. Be smarter.
    B. Love his mother more than his father.
    C. Grow up to be a heterosexual.
    D. Never go hungry.

4. Love means never having to say:
    A. "Shut up and go to bed."
    B. "Clean your room."
    C. "Leave me alone."
    D. None of the above.

5. If your child fails a math test in third grade, it means:
    A. Life is over. She sucks at math and will never get into MIT.
    B. You are a bad parent.
    C. Time to call in the tutor brigade.
    D. None of the above.

6. When your son's soccer coach doesn't start your son, you react by:
    A. Wondering aloud what you did to deserve this.
    B. Punching the coach in front of your son.
    C. Looking for another team.
    D. Enjoying the game.

7. When your daughter wins an award for the sixth-grade science fair, you:

   A. Tell her that you're proud of her.

   B. Hide the fact that you did her project for her.

   C. Hire a tutor to make sure that she maintains excellence in science.

   D. Tell her younger brother that you expect him to do the same next year.

8. Your child is not sure whether he wants to go to college. This make you feel:

   A. Worried. Can he get a good job these days without a college degree?

   B. Suicidal. His life will suck without going to college.

   C. Elated. College costs too much.

   D. Curious. Why does he feel that way?

9. If your son is being bullied by his seventh-grade classmates, what do you do?

   A. Intervene and ask questions later.

   B. Ignore it. After all, kids will be kids.

   C. Ask your son what's happening.

   D. Ask your spouse to take care of it.

10. When your five-year-old falls off a sliding board and breaks his arm, you choose to:

    A. Sue the inventor of the sliding board.

    B. Shrug and move on.

    C. Restrict his play activities for the next five years to the living room couch.

    D. None of the above.

Aptitude versus Fortitude

It's no surprise when we choose a piece of cake for dessert over a bunch of grapes. We know that the grapes are healthier and have their own good taste, but the cake—oh, my—the cake is just so sweet and satisfying, and considering all of our hard work, don't we deserve it?

It's a question of what we know versus what we feel, the ongoing struggle that we all face on a daily basis, whether it applies to our diets or how we parent our children.

"Oh, I should have known better!"

We often hear this response when regretting a choice that we've made, especially when it applies to something regarding our children. A recent *New York Times* article pointed out that parents who are able to defer gratification and control their impulses have children who become more successful. We all know this, yet we still often do what is easier, or what seems to make the child happier in the short run. When that happens, we probably have deep regrets and feel terrible, even for mild transgressions, yet we often continue doing the same thing.

Parenting inside this pressure cooker can force moms and dads of all shapes and stripes to overreact and do things triggered by their feelings or by expedience rather than by logic and good sense. This often begins when their children are very young. After all, these parents reason, if my kid is going to get a step ahead in life, it better start as soon as she learns how to walk!

From Playdates to Preschool: Too Much Programming

Nowadays, from the time children become toddlers, parents have a tendency to overprogram their schedules with an assortment of preschool activities, tutoring (yes, tutoring toddlers), after-preschool classes (yes, those, too), music appreciation, athletic activities, and an endless schedule of playdates. Parents probably take this route because they're worried that otherwise they might not be providing enough stimulation for their child, and their child will lag behind his or her peers when it really counts: later in life. After all, if your child can learn origami on Mondays, tae kwon do on Tuesdays, gymnastics on Thursdays, and dance on Fridays, and you can afford them all, how can a caring parent say no—particularly when some of your friends with kids the same age are doing them, too? Not to mention team sports and music lessons at least two or three days a week, before or after the other classes. Weekends, of course, are reserved for games, recitals, and tournaments. It's a wonder that your family even has time to sit down and eat, or watch your other children's activities.

Is all this necessary or even beneficial to children—at any age? It's nice to expose your kids to new ideas, new friends, and museums, but do they have to connect with all three every single day? Children need free time, downtime, do-nothing time, whatever you might call it—they need it. Parents need it, too. Imagine a day *without* racing around town from one activity to another. Someday, when your kids are grown and you are filling in as grandparents, you may appreciate the time you put in but also come to realize how much of it may have been extraneous, if not unnecessary.

To Schedule or to Chill?

Parents with demanding jobs that require them to put in long hours and/or travel out of town may feel guilty about being away from their children. As a result, they often overcompensate, either by overscheduling their kids with afterschool and weekend activities to make up for their lack of involvement, or by packing in too much activity during the parent-child time they *do* have, all in a misguided effort to make up for their limited time with their child. This is the same phenomenon that divorced parents who have their children only part-time go through when they try to package a week's worth of parenting into their limited visitation time.

For example, Mike, a caterer in a medium-sized New England suburb, works most weekends. When he finally has a Saturday off, he expects his children to be as ready and excited as he is to spend the entire day together, doing father-son and father-daughter things.

"Hey," he tells his kids, "we'll be best buddies this Saturday. We can go bowling, bike riding, and ice skating!"

Mike doesn't always take into account that his kids might have other plans for that Saturday and don't necessarily want to spend the entire day with their dad doing things. They may prefer staying home and doing not much of anything, but enjoying that time nevertheless because it's nice and relaxed and it's hanging out with their father.

But Mike insists.

"Hey, guys, I never get a Saturday off, and I want to *do* stuff with you guys. We're best buddies, after all, right?"

Mike's push to hyper-parent his kids may have a downside.

Child and family psychologist Richard Weissbourd, author of *The Parents We Mean to Be: How Well-Intentioned Adults Undermine Children's Moral and Emotional Development*, told Cristin Conger, author of *5 Signs of Overparenting*, that "we're the first parents in history who really want to be their kids' friends. Some parents even talk about wanting to be their kids' best friends."[1]

Weissbourd feels that when parents become so focused on bonding with their children, they may be sabotaging their own authority and doing so at the expense of traditional role modeling.

Because Mike is absent so often, he may not realize just how overscheduled his children are, and how much they need a break at least one day out of each weekend. By depriving his children of some necessary downtime, he takes away the chance for their creativity to flourish while their brains and bodies relax. Mike might also do himself a big favor by staying home to chill next time he has a Saturday free. You also want your children to be able to enjoy playing alone and have friends separate from you so that they will not spend all of their time just waiting for you to be available.

But What If?

Maybe Mike is right. Maybe his kids will be missing something if they don't bowl, ride bikes, and go ice-skating, particularly with him. Their friends may get better at those things, and that can't be good, can it? Plus, there's all that parent-child bonding that Mike has heard about, and if he wants to be as good a parent as his neighbors seem to be, with their camping trips and family barbecues, he better get busy.

Time-out. Are kids today more tightly scheduled than ever before because enrolling them in extracurricular activities and academic tutoring is considered a mark of highly effective and caring parents? Does "the busier the better" mean having more enriched lives or getting a step ahead of their friends on the way to résumé building for college? Do we all still believe that "idle hands do the devil's work?"

Maybe Mike's response should be, "OK, kids, go outside and play catch or whatever else you want to do." He might even start a trend among other parents.

"I didn't want to become the alpha-parent I kept seeing in the playground," says Tina, "fussing over their kids, directing who they played with and taking over the sandbox with their Neiman Marcus shoveling kit. I dreaded becoming that, but I began to feel guilty sitting on a bench twenty feet away, reading a magazine, and occasionally glancing over to make sure my kid was still playing and happy."

Unfortunately, Tina was falling into a trap that many others succumb to these days in this atmosphere of hyped-up parenting and an angst-driven need to succeed, one motivated by guilt and a fear that they may not be the ultimate parent, and in turn are letting their child down.

But what if Tina could just resist the temptation to become her worst nightmare? Would she and her daughter be happier?

It's worth remembering that our children are not our project, and as they become older, we must let them discover the world more and more on their own, with an appropriate amount of supervision. There lies the conundrum, the fuzzy line between too much supervision and safety and too little. How much supervision is enough, and when should we go further or sit back?

Do I Have to Wear a Helmet to Bed?

Parents with uncontrollable levels of anxiety about their children are prime candidates for overparenting. Where the parents' anxiety comes from is anybody's guess, but it's not terribly surprising to see parents worry themselves into a tizzy when it comes to the welfare of their kids. But this can have adverse effects on their children. At the first sign of a child's distress—for example, when they are learning to walk, ride a bike, or drive a car—moms and dads who are overanxious may suffocate their child with their own unreasonable concerns. In these cases, children can become as anxious as their parents, which will only increase their struggles and chance of failure.

An insistence on protecting your child at any cost is clearly counterproductive. Parents in these extreme situations overcompensate for whatever their own reasons are, and in essence generate more anxiety, which only leads to more worrying rather than normalizing.

What can follow is a move from anxiety to pure fear. For example, some parents will not allow their children to play outside without strict supervision because they are afraid that their children will be stolen. Even inside the house, they take protective measures to ensure that none of their children can possibly get bumped or bruised when playing. This goes past the point of just closing off electric sockets for infants, and moves on to covering sharp edges on tables and making sure that all floors have carpets for when the child falls, which they are apt to do. When parents behave to this extreme as their children grow up, it leaves them no flexibility to find a happy medium with more complicated issues, like how to let their children use modern-day communications.

As children begin to play, this vigilance is followed up with rubber-cushioned playgrounds (sadly preferred to grass, which can be dirty and theoretically have worse germs); a steady slathering of sanitizing gel whenever they go out, come in, or do something in between; and a large basketful of car seats, helmets, and body pads for miscellaneous activities. Some say that all of these safety devices are just a calculation by the manufacturers of these products to increase their profits by first creating panic among parents and then nurturing it with a continual series of studies proving how dangerous life is without suitable protection.

We want our children to be safe, whether it's at home, in school, or in between. Their physical well-being is of paramount importance, as is as their emotional and psychological health. But when do parents concerned for their child's safety become overprotective?

Techno Wars

With all the devices and diversions our children have at their disposal, it's no surprise that parents feel compelled to referee their kids' impulse to tweet, text, and otherwise plug in to a world of music, selfies, and video clips. The explosion of cell phone and Internet technology over the past twenty years has significantly altered contemporary parenting. All of the mobile devices currently available make it possible for parents to stay in contact with their children around the clock, even texting each other in the middle of the night from their respective bedrooms.

But is that always a good thing? Should parents become a family version of the NSA, spying on their own children? A few years ago, Taser, better known for making stun guns, introduced software that could intercept phone calls, text messages, and emails that are transmitted through personal cell phone use.[2] This extends an open invitation for parents to enter the surveillance business, with their children posing as their primary targets. Then there are all the possibilities that GPS technology offers, from live monitoring of a person's movement, even at preschool, to tracking their minute-by-minute location. Back on the home front, parents can use a number of different apps to monitor their children while they are alone or with a babysitter. This sort of technology can also provide police with up-to-date information and photos in the case of missing children.[3]

No one could argue with the benefits of this technology, especially if it protects children and in some cases saves their lives, but can keeping electronic tabs on our kids also have the opposite effect on both parents and children? Keeping our children on electronic leashes may very well alienate the very ones we are trying to protect. What ever happened to trust and teaching responsibility? It shouldn't be surprising that normal teenagers, who really have not been in any significant trouble, resent being followed and/or tracked—like a potential criminal—by their parents. Statistics show that crime rates have gone down nationwide during this generation, so parents in most cities and towns should appreciate this fact and give their kids the age-appropriate freedoms they deserve.[4]

Which Parents Are Most Susceptible to Overparenting?

Single parents, divorcees, widowers, high-achievers, stay-at-home parents, two-parent couples, type-A personalities, parents of adopted kids, low-income parents trying to make sure that their kids get a fair shake, same-sex parents, parents of gay children, and so forth—the list could go and on, meaning that anyone and everyone can join the crowd of parents who may just be trying too hard. Here is a sampling of parental types ripe for overparenting.

1. Dual-income households with expendable cash to devote to special activities for children.

In middle- and upper-class families all over the world, parents are obsessed with packing their children's lives full of a succession of activities from morning till night, with even more crammed into the weekends. In some communities, there seems to be a race going on to see which families are spending the most on their kids.

Julie, a mother in Hong Kong with a son and daughter who attend prestigious local schools, shared her excitement with the Rockmom.com's Ata Johnson about making a trip to Italy with her children over the summer holidays. She claimed that it would be their "last hurrah," a chance for her son, especially, to enjoy one last carefree summer before attending a fancy, all-boys school. Julie's son is seven.[5]

2. Parents working longer hours, who use extracurricular activities as a convenient option for childcare.

In his book *Under Pressure: Rescuing Our Children from the Culture of Hyper-Parenting*, author Carl Honoré says, "Now, everything is supervised, scheduled, controlled, and there's this strange unwillingness to let go or to be uncertain of anything. I think parents particularly want a single recipe for raising an alpha child, and there's a lot of pressure."[6]

Kevin, a high school freshman in Wichita, Kansas, complains about never getting a night off from the grind of homework.

"My parents freak out if I tell them I don't have any homework," he says. "They email my teachers to make sure I'm not lying and then make me study random stuff, just because I'm supposed to be learning, or whatever. I never get a night off."

In fact, many parents can't relax at all around the subject of homework. In a 2013 survey conducted by the homework resource website AskKids, 43 percent of the 778 parents asked admitted to having done their kids' homework at least once, to curb the stress their children were feeling.[7]

But are parents to blame when children feel overwhelmed by homework? We should look at schools and examine individual teachers to get a more accurate view of the matter.

"What would happen if we stopped helping our kids with homework?" asks Meg, a mother of three from Las Vegas, Nevada. "Our kids would get in trouble at school and probably be punished if they didn't hand in their homework. Then they would feel bad and get very grumpy."

Homework is a contentious subject in many households and school districts.

"A large body of existing research indicates that homework does not play an important role in student achievement," says Robert, a school board member from Missouri. "Apparently, it doesn't stimulate independence, either, or responsibility, and nothing proves that it builds character. Plus, it makes it really tough for kids with limited ability and resources. The research says so! The hype for more home-work is a myth! So, I would like to see a revision of our school district's homework policy."

Deciding the merits of homework does not rest entirely on the shoulders of parents. Much of it comes from school boards as well as teachers, and if parents want to make life infinitely more livable for their families, they should consider joining movements in their area that are fighting to reduce the amount of homework that schools are currently demanding of their children.

3. **Moms and dads who come to parenting later in life and bring a "time-is-running-out" or corporate mentality into the household. These parents tend to professionalize parenting by employing consultants and experts to ensure that their children will have the best of everything.**

Maybe this sums it up best:

Q: How many kids does it take to screw in a light bulb?

A: Is that with or without a tutor?

4. **The Joneses (see "keeping up with . . ."): these parents just can't help it.**

"I know that it's wrong to overprogram my kids," says Vicky, a mom of three in Boston, Massachusetts, "but if I don't, I feel inadequate as a parent. It's like I have to enroll them in as many extracurricular activities as their friends."

Parents put pressure on other parents to produce "all-star" children.

"Love to talk," says Jessica, a mother of two in Sacramento, California, "but I've got to go pick up my daughter Crystal at school and take her directly to ballet class—you know, the new one in town, it's so prestigious—and then she's got her French tutor—we meet her at Le Pain, you know that French café, it's so authentic there—and then we're racing off to join her synchronized swimming team. They're doing a charity performance at the country club, and I'm going to send photographs of Crystal to the US Olympic committee, because she'll be old enough in 2020 to join them! I'm sorry, am I going too fast?"

5. Parents who just aren't cut out for playing with their kids, so they hire people to do it for them.

An older, very wealthy father of a ten-year-old boy was known to have a teenager pick up his son to go play tennis with him at the father's country club because the father did not want to play, and did not want to join in with his son.

6. Safety nerds who can't stop worrying about their children's safety and resort to almost any length to protect them.

They are not hard to find. Just visit a typical playground and you will probably observe a parent going overboard, trying to protect his or her child from just about anything they consider threatening, from sand in the sandbox to water in the water fountain.

On his 1999 album and HBO special, *You Are All Diseased*, George Carlin bemoans how preoccupied Americans can be about child safety. "What ever happened to natural selection?" he asks. "If a child swallows seven marbles, maybe we don't want him to reproduce."[8]

But overprotective parenting is really no joke. When parents are *too* safe, they do not let their children grow into confident and independent adolescents and adults.

American parents are not the only ones who are overprotective. Indian parents are becoming synonymous with overprotecting their kids. Ritu will not let her nine-year-old son ride the school bus in Delhi because she has heard that the bus drivers are sometimes erratic. Sanji does not allow his thirteen-year-old daughter to have any sleepovers at her friends' houses because he's not confident that the other parents will provide adequate supervision. Priti gets so nervous when her seven-year-old son plays on a jungle gym in Calcutta that she won't let him do it by himself without standing right near him every step of the way. She will not allow her teenage daughter to go on a school picnic at the beach because she is afraid that her daughter may drown.[9]

7. Families with fewer children, who have more time to invest—literally—in each child.

Allison, a college placement counselor in an academically competitive high school, is always amazed by how quickly her phone calls to parents get returned. She feels like she has a red phone at the White House. When one dad returned her call, she heard an odd noise in the background.

"What's that noise?" she asked.

"Oh, it's nothing," said the dad on the line. "I can talk. I'm just doing a colonoscopy."

Allison didn't feel comfortable continuing the conversation and asked to call back later. The father—and devoted colonoscopy provider—insisted on continuing the conversation because, after all, it had something to do with his son, and what could possibly be more important than that?

Allison referred the father to a local parenting group that focuses on reprioritizing our values as parents.

8. Parents who send their kids to private schools and get anxious about everything once the first bill arrives in their mailbox.

Investing in our children can be taken too far, as evidenced by the following story.

A very exclusive, expensive, well-regarded, and academically rigorous international school in Hong Kong was planning to open a sister school on the mainland. The Hong Kong school planned to send their tenth-year students there for a year of study. The parents were split evenly as to whether that was a good idea. The most common objection: Homesickness? No. Parents missing their children? No. Most of the parents were worried about their children being away from their *tutors*.[10]

9. Immigrant parents raising their first child in America, who will do almost anything to help the child get ahead.

Families come to America from all over the world with the promise of free education and endless opportunities. But these immigrant parents aren't playing around. Citing the sacrifices they have made to come here, they put tremendous pressure on their children to succeed academically at the highest level. Luckily, many of these families come from countries with a strong work ethic, so their children do excel in school.

When American-born parents realize that their children's futures are threatened by this "foreign" competition, they often react with fear and anxiety, not only by pushing their children unreasonably, but by intervening on their behalf, succumbing to the worst of what overparenting can become.

Both sets of parents, the native-born and the newly arrived, essentially turn their children's lives into a series of hurdles to jump over and through in order to finish first in a race to what they consider to be the top.

10. Parents with an abstract fear of failure.

In Colorado Springs, Colorado, organizers of an annual Easter egg hunt attended by hundreds of children canceled last year's event, citing the behavior of aggressive parents who swarmed into the tiny park the previous year, determined that their kids get an egg.[11]

Was it pure greed that drove these parents to act so badly? Let's hope not, because unless there was an acute shortage of Easter eggs in Colorado going on at the time, such a thing is unfathomable. Was it guilt? How much guilt were these parents possibly feeling that they had to fight over Easter eggs?? Were they all trying to fix something in their kids' lives that only a painted egg could accomplish? Most likely they did not want their child to feel bad or be the one kid who did not find an egg or who got the smallest number of eggs in his or her basket to take home. Once again, here is an instance of parents trying to protect their children from a perceived sense of failure.

A Warning to Divorcing Parents

If you are a parent in the midst of a divorce or somewhere in the aftermath of that process, chances are that you are very susceptible to overparenting, simply because you can't help feeling as if you are competing with your ex for the affections of your children.

Because divorce has become more common over the past two or three decades, often played out in public, children are increasingly caught in the middle of their parents' bad behavior. These parents just can't help themselves when it comes to contesting and competing about everything, including what they do with their children, which invariably leads to overparenting by both parties. Divorce attorneys joke about these "Super Dads" and "Super Moms," who often are also trying to improve their position in front of the judge to impact the amount of visitation—and, in turn, the money—either party will pay out or receive.

Sadly, these conflicted moms and dads, wrenched apart from their children for days and/or weeks at a time, are quick to lose the good judgment they formerly possessed. This plays out during their one-on-one time with their children, when they try to score points with their kids by being "the better parent." This often means trying to ensure that the child has a good time with them, doing what the child wants, and providing almost no discipline for the child, so that they will want to come back and be with them during the next weekend or holiday.

If that is what you are doing, only bad things will happen. Divorce is hard, no matter how amicably it is conducted. If you are used to being with your children on a daily basis, and then you are stripped of that privilege by the agreement you arrange with your ex, those lonely days and nights without them can not only make you hurt, they can shake your confidence and lead you to say things and act out in ways you may regret. Disparaging the other parent is one way to do that, while overindulging your child is another.

If you are feeling vulnerable to all that, seek help to keep your balance.

Communication Gaps May Lead to Overparenting

In families coping with a divorce, parents and children face increased levels of stress, complete with varying degrees of denial, guilt, and confusion. As a result, communication between parents and children may suffer at a time when it really is most important and necessary. This irony of how parents and children view the effects of divorce differently and their inability to communicate about it is best illustrated by the following study.

When a parenting website in the United Kingdom[12] surveyed one thousand parents and one hundred children (separately) about divorce, they discovered that 39 percent of the kids said that they hide their feelings about the split from their parents, 20 percent said that there's no use communicating because their parents are too "wrapped up in themselves," and 14 percent said that they couldn't be honest with their parents about how upset they felt. Nearly one-third of kids under eighteen described themselves as "devastated" by the divorce, and 13 percent blamed themselves for their parents' breakup.

On the other hand, 77 percent of the parents expressed confidence that their kids were dealing just fine with the divorce. Ten percent thought that their kids were relieved that their parents had split. But only 5 percent of parents were aware of their children's blaming themselves for the situation. Even more alarming, only 1 percent of the parents knew about their kids' resorting to alcohol, self-harm, and contemplating suicide as a reaction to their parents' divorce.

While these statistics alone do not point to parental problems, it's not surprising that the trauma of divorce can lead parents, fueled by guilt, to overcompensate, often without even being aware of it. The study also points out that it is very important to talk to your children and to listen to what they say, even if you don't always want to hear it. Clearly, these parents had their own agendas, and didn't ask their children, didn't listen when the kids told them what they didn't want to hear, or simply minimized what they were told to fit into their own view of the situation.

Who Are You Really Helping?

It's clear from these parental subgroups that all of us are susceptible to overparenting. We want the best for our children, and most of us will occasionally overparent, especially during times of crisis. We don't want anyone to cut in line during our children's march to the top, and we are ready to protect them and advocate for them every step of the way. It all sounds good, until we consider the consequences of all that attention, protection, and advocacy.

Stephen Asma, professor of philosophy and distinguished scholar at Columbia College in Chicago, sums up the moral conflict for parents in his 2012 book *Against Fairness*.

"If some science-fiction sorcerer came to me with a button and said I could save my son's life by pressing it but then (cue the dissonant music) ten strangers would die somewhere . . . I'd have my finger down on it before he finished his cryptic challenge."[13]

As far as hyper-competitive parents are concerned, in the ultra-competitive world we live in, the choices we make on behalf of our kids boil down to one thing: survival of the fittest.

"It *is* a jungle out there," according to Suzi, a parent of four from Brooklyn, New York, who spoke to us last year. "Either my kid gets into that great school or into the starting line-up of the fifth grade volleyball team or somebody else's will, and that could mean the difference between Harvard University and the local community college."

While Suzi may mean well, becoming so invested in our children—emotionally, psychologically, and financially—can make us do strange and harmful things—to ourselves and to them. It might be wise to reconsider our behavior. Not every child is destined for the Ivy League, and some kids may be better off somewhere else. For some kids, a community college, especially during their first year or two after high school, when they have no idea what they want to study or do with their lives, is not an unreasonable idea. For parents looking to spend their money wisely, this might be a sensible path to consider. It is also important to recognize the fact that many very successful people in terms of personal happiness, financial success, and a fulfilling family life have attended community college and non–Ivy League institutions.

Fighting the Odds

In today's parenting world, it's not easy to avoid overdoing it, especially when you consider everything parents must navigate while trying to do the best for their child. From the pressure to enroll your child in a good school to the constant lure of texting, not to mention tutoring companies and the steep mountain that parents are told they must climb to ensure their child a prime spot in college, mothers and fathers face a battle of wills when it comes to resisting the pull to overparent.

So, when you screw up, which is inevitable, at least sometimes, it may not be your fault at all. Just as succumbing to peer pressure was easy when you were a youth, it remains challenging as an adult, especially if you have even a hint of anxiety about yourself and your child's ability to keep up with his or her peers. Everywhere you turn, you are assaulted by come-ons, telling you what you need to do in order to attain that edge for your kid.

It is almost as if we need a twelve-step program for parents who can't control themselves, or an Al-Anon type of program to try to stop saving our children. Once again, it boils down to being smart, letting go, and making sure that you have a life of your own, independent of your child's.

The temptation is everywhere. Parenting self-help books (like this one!) are conveniently located right next to children's books in the stores, and you can find even more of them online. Some schools offer parents the chance to download their child's grades every day so that they can post them on the refrigerator at home or on Facebook. "Save Your Family" workshops are advertised in every local and regional parenting magazine, and national publications never stop telling you what you are doing wrong, what you are (almost) doing right, and what new magical advice exists to make parenting an instantly more rewarding experience for you and your child. If you haven't been knocked out by now, college recruiters, testing companies, and a still-growing tutoring industry are all competing for your bank accounts, not to mention private schools that are raising tuition each year and

PTAs that are hunting for donations. Add to this the scientific push to get everyone's performance enhanced with ADHD medication, and it's no surprise that there are many days when parents feel out of control. And it's no wonder that perfectly smart and capable parents leave their jobs and devote 100 percent of their lives to their kids, only to discover before too long that all the pressure drives them crazy, if not clinically neurotic, which no doubt will rub off quite quickly on their children.

CHAPTER 4: THE AGONY AND THE ECSTASY OF YOUR ACTIVE CHILD

Mothers and fathers from Kentucky to California are obsessed with their children's athletic endeavors. You can see them at basketball games, soccer matches, and volleyball tournaments, holding up giant posters of their child, cheering so loudly that other people attending the games may need to ask them to pipe down, reminding them that their child is not the only one competing. Some parents can become so "enthusiastic" that their behavior—considered by them to be simply supportive—can get them thrown out of the gym.

Some parents are so hungry for their children to excel in their chosen sport because it can be the ticket to a college education. These parents have been known to switch their children from one school to another, searching for the optimum situation that will guarantee their child the most playing time and opportunity for college scouts to see them play.

All across the country, these fierce moms and obsessive dads are taking the idea of supportive parenting to a level of hysteria and stress perhaps never seen before. YouTube is teeming with video clips of children as young as four or five years old, dribbling a soccer ball the length of the field and scoring against another child playing goalie who may not be even facing the incoming ball at the time of the shot, being more interested at the age of four in a passing squirrel near the field.

These parents are posting video clips not because their child is so cute. It's because they think their child is so *good* at a particular sport that the recruiting process should begin before the child is barely out of diapers and continue as he or she grows, ratcheting up to a fever pitch by the time the child is in high school.

All of these anxious, promotion-crazed parents have one thing in common: they want their sons and daughters to be good enough to earn a scholarship to college, and they see sports as the ticket. But pushing this so hard does not always go over so well with other parents, their children's coaches, and even their sons and daughters.

For single parents working multiple jobs, an athletic scholarship may be the only way they imagine that they can send their child to a university. So when these parents attend games, they tend to get carried away. We see multiple instances of parents getting into fights in bleachers and losing control during timeouts, cajoling coaches to play their child more. It can get so bad that security officers are needed to escort these overactive parents out of the gym.

Sounds like a perfect scene for reality TV and it wouldn't be surprising if we see something like that one day on our screens. We can laugh at the prospect of a show called *Basketball Moms and the Kids They Humiliate* but shouldn't we be considering the children in these cases? How do these children feel when their parents act out publicly in such a manner? Generally, kids will not enjoy that type of behavior, especially in front of their friends and fellow players.

But many parents persist, pushing their kids to play year-round at tournament after tournament, with special coaching on the side, meaning in some cases that, academic studies become sacrificed for the chase after athletic dreams.

Whose dreams are these, really, and what will happen if these "rising stars" don't make it? Because of their focus on sports—often exclusively—many of these kids have devoted little time to schoolwork and will be lucky to get into a community college at best. It's not surprising that many of them become resentful of their parents because of all the missed social events and leisure-time activities with peers. Without those experiences to develop social skills and a general sense of self-reliance, these kids are poorly prepared to move on with life after what they can only consider to be their first major failure in life. Sadly, because they have learned few, if any, coping mechanisms for disappointment while growing up, drugs and alcohol beckon easily as a convenient alternative.

Like It or Not

Just as we can't predict how our children will turn out, we don't always know what we're getting into when we introduce our children to the world of youth sports. We know that developing athletic skills in a team context can help a child build self-confidence while learning to relate to and share with others. But these days, even a recreational league can be pretty intense and may present our children with a much more competitive agenda than we bargained for. While some coaches are friendly parents, glorified "cupcake providers" if you will, who know little more about the game than the kids and just want to make sure that every kid has a uniform and plays equal time, other adults take the game much more seriously. They often put the children in a precarious position, where winning is everything and an individual child's self-esteem and feelings are unimportant. For these coaches, the goal is not to make the children feel better about themselves while developing a skill and socializing; it's winning for the coach, under the guise of winning for the team, sometimes at any cost.

You'll recognize those parent volunteers because they will remind you of the middle school bully who shoved around other kids on the playground and pushed girls into the fence if they didn't give him the attention he wanted. Now, all grown-up with children of their own, these men (mostly) are the ones who have chosen to be responsible for teaching their kids as well as yours the merits of fair play, teamwork, and, coincidentally, how to throw a ball.

Watch out: these coaches, dads *and* moms, will go to extremes to win. Against league rules dictating equal playing time for everybody, they will fudge substitution patterns so that their best athletes will play the most minutes. They will rudely challenge referees and umpires in full view of their young players, setting an atrocious example for the children to whom they are supposed to be teaching good sportsmanship. And, because they have not yet fully realized that they've already graduated from high school many years ago and that their athletic careers are over, they will do whatever it takes to win the game, even if it means cheating or bending the rules to show up their fellow parent-coaches.

According to a study of more than five hundred students at the Los Angeles–based Josephson Institute, student athletes can be some of the most dishonest kids. The institute found that more than 72 percent of football players admitted to having cheated during various examinations. Where does this attitude come from? The study suggests that it might be from the coaches.[1]

How does what is supposed to be skill building and character development come to this? In today's era, where pressure on parents to help their child get ahead is overwhelming, and parents are constantly afraid that their kids might fail (which means that *they* as parents have failed, too), anything is fair play, and that applies to almost any arena. These parents, motivated by anxiety and desperation, will push to try to make anything happen for the benefit of their child. In previous generations, sports were not organized with any adult supervision until high school. Parents attended games or other events only when they could get time off from work and when the games or events were extremely important. Otherwise, parents and children shared their athletic endeavors in the backyard with a simple game of catch.

Performance Isn't Everything

While it may not always be the most athletic thing to witness, what's better than watching a father and son play catch in the backyard or, even better, alone on the local diamond, pretending like they're participating in a crucial World Series game? It's heartwarming to watch a parent and child bond as something remarkably comforting and reassuring takes place for them during a simple game of catch. You throw a ball to someone else, wait a sec, and it comes back! Every time! Or it pretty much does, if your dad has half an arm, which when you're a kid, he certainly seems to. In fact, for most young boys and girls, playing catch is like a perfect moving security blanket, with each toss representing something you can trust in the world. When you throw the ball, that treasured possession that you imagine you might never part with, you are going to get it back! The person you trust most in the world continues to win your love because he—or she—simply throws it back! That person is spending time with you, teaching you, showing you that he is not perfect, because he occasionally drops the ball or mis-throws it, but with each toss and catch, you feel like an absolute winner, and that's all that matters! As a parent, you also feel like a winner because you are doing something important with your child besides just teaching them how to play catch.

So what happens to those moms and dads who end up overparenting courtside, on the ball field, from the audience, or at home in the backyard? How did they get to the point of harassing everyone in sight, simply because their child is so important—to *them*? Is it just the prospect of a college scholarship? Is it a sense that because they are so important, their child must be as well? For some parents, like the ones at the beginning of this chapter, this is all the rationale they need to push, push, push and let the chips fall where they will. But for many other parents, especially those who can afford college tuitions (and paying back loans), why are they pushing their kids so hard? Why are they cheering so loud? Do they really think that their child is the only one on the field or in the musical? Is it the fact that they consider their child to be an extension of them, and, in some cases, that the child may be making up for the parent's own imperfections?

Whether your son or daughter is a fledgling student athlete, actor, dancer, or chess player, he or she has unique reasons for participating in whatever activity he or she chooses. Or has the child chosen? Some parents enroll their children in theater, music, or dance lessons—and sometimes all of them—without much thought for their child's preferences. They view it simply as something their child should do to be cultured, well-rounded, and a better candidate down the road for life, which also means acceptance at what ultimately may be a prestigious university. Some parents even hire private coaches to supplement their child's regularly scheduled practice regimen, again to give them a leg up on everyone else.

The upshot of all this is that many children are spending too much time in isolated activities, such as piano lessons (with its requisite solitary practice hours), or in *supervised* team sports, where every minute of every practice and game is watched by coaches, referees, and a ubiquitous squad of parents.

Karen, a mom with two kids from Atlanta, Georgia, describes a seemingly new option for parents whose children may not be athletically or artistically inclined. These parents would prefer to not waste any time developing their children's other talents and jump right to the top.

"When a parent I know recently recommended a class to me that offers to train your child to develop executive skills, I thought I might be sick. My son is six! He plays with LEGO. He doesn't have to run their company. He can do that when he's nine. I'm kidding. Really, if you have little kids, why can't we just let them relax and enjoy their childhood? It only lasts a short time. Once they become teenagers, they are sucked in to getting into college and become adults, and that means for *the rest of their lives,* so I told that parent I would be skipping the executive training class for my son and that she should just go home and get a life."

Kids need free time for unstructured play. Consider it to be an educational moment. And if you need someone to give you permission to let your kids do that, or if you require a prescription with instructions to back off and let your child be a child, feel free to use this book as your ticket to do so. Play is a simple human interaction, a joyful alternative to the essential conundrum that we human beings face each day. Unfortunately, most adults forget that after they have passed through childhood. But if a child does not learn to play, to entertain himself and take pleasure in what he does when he is little, he will never learn it when he is older. As humans we are intrinsically selfish but also biologically social. While we thrive on cooperating with others, we are also always looking out for ourselves. Finding that balance is what children do every day, at home with their siblings and at recess with their friends. Let them. Let them be kids!

The best thing parents can do is back off and let their kids figure out things for themselves, just like they probably did when they were children. Remember "benign neglect"? If your child needs help, he or she will come and talk with you.

The Curse of Electronics and the War of the Thumbs

Back in the day, when someone was said to have a "green thumb," it meant that he or she was adept at gardening and other functions related to Mother Earth. We hardly ever hear that phrase anymore, certainly not from anyone under the age of twenty-one, whose response might be, "You have a green thumb? Huh? What, is your cell phone green, and it's, like, leaking its color onto your thumbs when you text?"

While this comment may demonstrate a certain knack for deductive thinking in our era, it also illustrates how constricted and single-minded most children are today as they grow up glued to their phones and other communication devices.

"It's not a question of free time," says Molly, a mother of four in Portland, Oregon. "My youngest kids—and many others I know—have tons of free time, but they hardly ever use it to play outside. I think you have to take modern culture and technology into account. Most kids these days will choose TV or video games over actual playing with other kids. They'd rather stay inside playing video games or doing stuff on their iPhones. I've tried to curb these things with my kids, but when other kids come over to play, this is what they all want to do. This is a tremendous problem facing our society, but it's not really a school issue, and it's not exactly a parent issue. It's just what our whole world is moving into, and I don't know how to stop it."

Molly is not alone. Many parents rue the day that they caved in and bought their adolescent kids a cell phone. Sure, it makes communication easier, but at what price? Most of us would prefer that our children spend less time indoors interacting with electronic devices and more time outside, interacting with each other and nature. Even children as young as two or three years old can get their hands on one of their parent's smartphones, which are loaded up with games they can play whenever they have a free moment, be it at home or even sitting in a restaurant, waiting for lunch.

But not everyone necessarily agrees that electronic devices prevent or inhibit social interaction and social development. Susan Kuhn, a technology futurist and digital strategist in Arlington, Virginia, told Michael De Groot of the *Deseret News* that fear is behind much of the opposition to smartphones and allowing kids to have them.[2]

"Information technology is evolving faster than anything in human history," Kuhn told De Groot. "The key is to not just look at the device, but the role it is playing."

The attraction of new technology is obvious. Kids can create websites and make videos in the palm of their hand, share them in an instant, pass around other cool things of interest, and expand their learning options anywhere they are—at school, at home, or on the road.

"Smartphones are going to be very important in the future," said Kuhn in the same article by De Groot. "Parents should want their children to master the tool and use it well. Kids are going to grow up in a world of instant communication and ubiquity of information. We do right by our children when we help them to grow up able to live in the world that is coming for them, the world of the future—not the world where we are comfortable, the world of what we grew up in."

Is it too late for children today to learn how to balance technology with life away from connectivity and commercial stimulation? Has that ship already sailed, or can parents still balance their children's use of electronic devices with exposure to nature and physical activity? Perhaps the newest wave of parents will work a little harder to introduce their first-born toddlers to the magic of the great outdoors, starting with their own backyards or local parks.

Louis C. K. Explains Why He Doesn't Want His Kids to Have Smartphones

Electronic devices help people escape from themselves and their feelings, particularly the sad or unhappy ones. It is often after a period of loneliness or loss that we come to understand why we feel that way and come up with new, positive, and creative ways to deal with our underlying issues. Using electronic toys as a way to keep oneself stimulated is a way to avoid those feelings by pretending they are not really there. When we take that route, we never deal with them or move on in our life.

Comedian Louis C. K. once explained to Conan O'Brien exactly why he dislikes the culture of smartphones and why he would never get one for his kids. He starts off by suggesting that smartphone usage is the reason why kids today are meaner:

"I think these things are toxic," he told Conan, "especially for kids... they don't look at people when they talk to them, and they don't build empathy."[3]

Texting opens up the door to exchanging hurtful words and sentiments without any real-life confrontation, making it easier for bullying among children to exist. But smartphones also can effect grown-ups in negative ways, causing many of us to become obsessed with communicating with others and being "in touch" with everything going on around us—*all* the time.

Louis C. K. had his own take on the foibles of texting when he spoke to Conan.

"That's why we text and drive. I look around, pretty much 100 percent of the people driving are texting. And they're killing; everybody's murdering each other with their cars. But people are willing to risk taking a life and ruining their own because they don't want to be alone for a second, because it's so hard."

He's definitely got a point. All the technology, the capability for constant contact and stimulation, can keep us from ever having any authentic solitude and calm. It might be even worse for our children, who are growing up with no alternative. It's rare nowadays to see children, especially once they have a cell phone of their own, just hanging out *without* an electronic device in their hand. It's no wonder that kids today have a hard time just sitting still, doing nothing and letting life percolate inside them.

Don't we as parents need to help them settle in with solitary time, with the idea that sometimes each of us *is* alone and that like it or not, it's part of life? Can't we coax our children toward a place where they can experience their own feelings without having to distract themselves by incessantly texting a bunch of their friends?

In essence, what Louis C. K. is saying is that electronic devices can be a way to avoid dealing with your own feelings while avoiding real interactions with other people. Feelings, communication, and relationships are what we are all about as people, yet these devices help us avoid making genuine connections.

The Free-Play Challenge

Over the past two generations, children in the United States have been given less and less opportunity to enjoy free time and the wonderful realm of play it provides.

In *Children at Play: An American History*,[4] author Howard Chudacoff calls the first half of the twentieth century the "golden age" of free play for children.

After the initial surge of the Industrial Revolution, the need for child labor declined, so by the early 1900s children enjoyed their free time. But, gradually, children began to suffer a loss in their leisure time as adults began increasing how many hours were to be spent doing schoolwork. Along with that, parents were putting the clamps on their children's freedom to play on their own, even when school was out and their kids had no homework. Adult-directed sports began to replace pickup games and sandlot sports. Afterschool classes and tutorials began to replace hobbies.

To make matters worse, as crime rates rose, that meant that parents became afraid—rightfully so, in many cases—and began to keep their children from playing outside—unsupervised—with other kids. This mind-set hasn't changed very much, even as crime rates have declined in many areas. In fact, organized sports, arts programs, and afterschool academic activities have increased, leaving children with even less free time than ever.

Not coincidentally, diagnoses of childhood mental disorders have increased as children's free-play options have decreased. This is because we are seeing not just disorders that may have been previously missed or not diagnosed, but an increase in diagnostic categories that have remained consistent over that time. For example, since the 1950s, groups of average schoolchildren have been given the same clinical questionnaires aimed at assessing anxiety and depression. Analyses of the results over the past few decades reveal a continuous, essentially linear, increase in anxiety and depression in young people. The rates we see today of what would be appropriately diagnosed as generalized anxiety disorder and major depression are five to eight times what they were in the 1950s. Over the same period, the suicide rate for young people aged fifteen to twenty-four has more than doubled, and for children under age fifteen it has quadrupled.[5] There also is an increase in other diagnoses, such as ADHD, Asperger's syndrome, and bipolar disorder in children because the mental health profession has introduced a variety of different labels for kids who used to be seen as a little different but still fit in and were involved with everyone else. Now they are often labeled and put into specialized treatment or training programs.

This suggests that the benefits of free play for children are being pushed aside in favor of an increasing amount of hyper-scheduling on the part of parents. We must examine who benefits from this trend, both in the short run and long term. All of the privately funded companies providing services for families—from afterschool "study buddies" to Pee Wee football programs, from College Board test preparation institutions to music academies and dance studios—have created an industry worth billions in today's market. None of these businesses have any desire to see children have more free time. In fact, they would prefer exactly the opposite—more classes, more kids, more cash. In the public sector, public schools are fighting to provide more services for the families of their students, many of whom come from single-parent homes or families with two working parents, both of which need more daily hours of childcare.

Any way you slice it, kids today are being pushed to become more and more involved in a variety of different activities. The importance of it is seen—and sold—as a matter of improving the overall educational level of our children as well as a question of public health. With the rising rate of childhood obesity, it's no wonder that parents are being encouraged to enroll their kids in extracurricular sports activities. For parents who admit that their children have weight issues, this can be helpful, but why is free-play time not considered valuable even within this health-care equation? However, free-play time must be something other than having your children sitting in their rooms alone, playing on their computers or some other electronic gadgets.

What no one can dispute is that parents have become more and more vigilant about scheduling their children with more and more activities. How much is helpful, and when do the children become overloaded? When parents respond to other parents getting their kids involved in those same activities by signing up their own kids for even more things to do, this sets up a competitive atmosphere in which the question for parents becomes whose child can be involved in more activities, or are you a bad parent if you do not schedule your child for enough? Parents suspend their better judgment and get sucked into a vortex of signing their kids up for every available "special" opportunity, in the end depriving their children of the one thing they may need most: rest and relaxation.

Bullying: Defining Our Role as Parents

While children can surely benefit from unsupervised play and more recess time in school, both of these leisure activities can also invite bullying, and some of it can become quite vicious. Bullying itself is nothing new, but as our news outlets report on a constant basis, it seems like it has escalated and grown more intense. Cyber bullying plays a large role in that increase. Since emailing, texting, and social networking sites have become so prevalent, the amount of bullying seems to have increased exponentially. It used to be that when you went home after school, you were safe and protected from the school bully until the next day, but in today's electronic age, kids can never really get away from the threat of bullying. There is no escape, nowhere truly safe, unless someone shuts off your electricity.

"As a child, I can remember 'sticks and stones can break your bones, but words will never hurt you,'" says Sheriff Grady Judd of Polk County, Florida, who presided last year over the case of Rebecca Ann Sedwick, a twelve-year-old girl who committed suicide after a year of face-to-face and cyber bullying. "Today," the sheriff added, "words stick because they are printed and they are there forever."[6]

Schools, in particular, are trying to police this dangerous activity, but because most of it occurs outside school hours, it's quite difficult for them to be effective. However, schools can do something about the bullying that occurs on their own turf.

"Our children's elementary school recently began supervising organized sports during lunchtime," says April, a mother of two in Lansing, Michigan, describing her situation to us. "Instead of the kids hanging around all that time with little supervision, which definitely made it easy for bullying to happen, the atmosphere now has really improved, and many children are enjoying school a lot more because of this administrative change."

But what about the role of parents in thwarting bullying? Dieter Wolke, PhD, professor of developmental psychology at The University of Warwick Medical School in the UK, thinks that overprotection by parents can increase the risk [that] a child will be bullied.[7] According to a recent study published in *Child Abuse & Neglect,* researchers conducted a meta-analysis of seventy studies on more than two hundred thousand children.

"Since parental support and supervision are important aspects to prevent bullying," Wolke reports, "the researchers were particularly surprised to find that overprotective parenting can have adverse effects on children. Parents who try too hard to buffer their children from harm, they assessed, can actually hurt them."

The goal of parenting, Dr. Wolke suggests, is to make children competent, self-regulating, and effective people. Just as we should not treat our children with antibiotics every time they have a sniffle, we also need to give them the chance to learn how they can deal with stress, albeit in appropriate doses. If they don't learn those small life lessons, they will have trouble when it comes to facing larger issues, like bullying.

Whether our child is being bullied or is the one *doing* the bullying, should we intervene, and, if so, when and how, and how much? It's a tough call and practically impossible to generalize, but it does appear that overprotective parenting tends to develop children who in turn are more vulnerable or susceptible to being bullied. What might seem like bullying to one child might just be some harmless razzing to another. It's a question of age, environment, number of siblings, the child's place in the birth order, and subtle shifts in subcultures. Parental support can come in many ways besides overprotection or intervention. One middle schooler who was continually being bullied, and revealed as much to his parents, was told that the only way to stop it was to punch the bully. While he was smaller than the bully, he did it anyway, and it ended, although the two children never did move on to become friends. This was more effective than the parents' stepping in to intervene for the child or getting the bully's parents involved, who are often bullies themselves.

Because some people in our society have become more accepting of racial, religious, and sexual differences, children (as well as adults) are interacting with each other with more tolerance and support. But there could be a lot more, as demonstrated by the amount of bullying that still exists. In fact, it's not just the immediate effects of bullying that should concern us. In many cases, it can have lasting effects.

According to *The New York Times*, Catherine P. Bradshaw, an expert on bullying and deputy director of the Center for the Prevention of Youth Violence at Johns Hopkins University, says that, "the experience of bullying in childhood can have profound effects on mental health in adulthood, particularly among youths involved in bullying as both a perpetuator and a victim."[8]

A study of the long-term effects of bullying in school, published in February 2013 in the journal *JAMA Psychiatry*, shows that victims and bullies alike can experience a heightened risk of trouble lasting well into adulthood.[9]

"We were actually able to say being a victim of bullying is having an effect a decade later, above and beyond other psychiatric problems in childhood and other adversities," said William E. Copeland, lead author of the study and an associate professor of psychiatry and behavioral sciences at Duke University Medical Center. "The pattern we are seeing is similar to patterns we see when a child is abused or maltreated or treated very harshly within the family setting."

The evidence presented is rather daunting and worthy of our attention, but the reality of what can happen with our children right here and now—especially from the rash of cyber bullying that is happening—is far more troubling.

With new apps popping up so frequently, it's very difficult for parents to keep up with the social platforms and photo-sharing applications that their children are using. This is especially true with adolescent children, whose newly emerging independence must be, at the very least, acknowledged, if not respected. So how do parents know when to get involved? And what's too much or too little?

Sheriff Judd in Florida puts it best: "Watch what your children do online. Pay attention. Quit being their best friend and be their best parent. That's important."

"I Coulda Been a Contenduh"

"The first place we must look for the origins of bullying is the behavior of parents," Mrs. Brando says, addressing her classroom of adults. Mrs. Brando treats parents who have been arrested on misdemeanor charges for acting out against other parents, teachers, or coaches for reasons connected to their own children.

"It's not hard to find parents trying to intimidate their children's teachers or even fighting with their child's coaches," she continues. "Some of these parents are clearly in need of a good parenting class, if not formal treatment."

"Yeah, I know," chimes in Trent, a former semiprofessional hockey player, who until recently was coaching his son in a Pee Wee league for six-year-olds. "It means our kids make us really bummed out one minute, like when they fall down on the ice instead of scoring, and then they make us, like, really happy when they do something right, like win the game."

"Exactly!" barks Mrs. Brando (no relation to Marlon), who, judging by the bulge in her eyes, is obviously unhappy with the reaction of her class. "You, Trent, and most of the rest of you in here, have managed to make everything in your life revolve around your child and how it reflects on you. Let's begin with mistake number one. For example, when it comes to young children playing a game on ice while skating on blades the thickness of a kitchen knife, we should realize that they will fall, and quite often. So, why, Trent, knowing how difficult it can be to skate at high speeds while trying to corral a moving puck, did you storm onto the ice last week and start screaming at your son just because he missed a shot and got his skate stuck in the netting of the goal? And then what prompted you to slug the referee when he tried to intervene?"

"Now, you don't understand," Trent says. "You don't know what it's like to be a former big-time hockey player watching his own flesh and blood mess up on the ice right there in front of you and a whole bunch of their kids and their parents. It's downright embarrassing. I mean, when he messes up, he makes me look like a loser!"

"Excuse me, Trent," Mrs. Brando interrupts. "Are you telling me that when your six-year-old son slips and falls on the ice while he's speeding around trying not to crash into anybody while carrying a big stick, he's messing up? And as a former semiprofessional hockey player, you consider that a reflection on you, is that right? You find it humiliating? Yes? Did I get that right?"

Trent looks around the room, nodding, looking for approval from his peers, and turns back to Mrs. Brando.

"Uh, I guess so, yeah; it's a rough world out there."

"Well, Trent," Mrs. Brando continues, "I don't think it's necessary to point out how foolish that sounds, but I do suppose there's one good thing about your reaction to your son when he falls down. You obviously let him get back up on his own, which is the only evidence of good parenting I can see in this whole fiasco."

"Mrs. Brando," Trent begins, "are you trying to tell me that I should stay on the bench and let my kid screw up like the other kids? Huh? Is that what you're telling me?"

"Very good, Trent, you're learning—at your own pace, but still. As for the rest of you, same time next week. And please, give your kids a break and stay out of trouble."

Whatever Happened to Pickup Ball?

In the process of trying to become a contender for Parent of the Year, or trying to turn your child into the Student Athlete of the Year, many parents put way too much pressure on their children to perform at unrealistic and unsustainable levels. Competitive sports have their benefits in the exercise and lessons in teamwork they provide, but when parents drive their kids, like Trent does, they may turn off the child before he or she has even had the chance to reap the full benefits that sports provides. Unfortunately, as parents of star T-ball players and preschool soccer stars find out, when children's sports are adult-directed by parents, as is the case with Trent, children often burn out and lose interest before they get to high school.

Why is that? During a typical school day, adults are guiding children through nearly every aspect of their lives and their learning. Many parents assume that their children will also function well *after* school and on weekends, particularly if adults again structure them and lead the way. It is as if the kids would be totally lost or would be latchkey kids if no one constantly told them what to do. The problem is that many kids today are never left alone to their own devices to organize their own teams and play their own games, and to stop playing when they want. They don't have enough free time or free choice! The parents' feelings of guilt and pressure to be "perfect" too often lead them to fill their children's every waking moment with activities, complete with someone hovering over the children to be sure that they "do it right." The parents' concern is that if their children are out of their sight (or another responsible adult's) or given the chance to decide things for themselves, which of course includes arguing and eventually reconciling, they won't be successful, or do anything to further their chances for "advancement." At the first hint of conflict, too many parents intervene, as if a little turmoil is harmful to children's health.

"I went to school in the seventies," says Kim, from Fairfax, Virginia. "I took music classes and played softball every spring while the boys played baseball. There were no travel teams or coaches back then, which would have obligated us kids to participate all year-round, even if we didn't want to sometimes. Instead, we gathered in our neighborhood most of the time, all mixed ages, shapes, and sizes, and we picked up teams for whatever sport was in season, argued, got angry with each other sometimes, and always figured out how to fix whatever problem we were having—by ourselves. Parents never got involved. Threats of 'I'm gonna tell your father!' were not taken seriously. Kids only resorted to that when they otherwise ran out of things to say. What would they tell him anyway, 'cause he was busy and just glad we were out of the house and doing something? We weren't all best friends, but we were totally cool without adult supervision. Does that even happen anymore? I don't think so."

Kim is right. Over the past twenty-plus years, the rise in organized afterschool activities and interscholastic competitive sports programs has spurred a frenzy of misplaced enthusiasm among parents who seem to think that their children are destined to play professional sports. But the number of student athletes who go on to play at a professional level is not only small; it's barely perceptible. However, that doesn't keep parents and schools from pumping more and more money into athletic programs, especially at secondary schools.

In "The Case Against High-School Sports,"[10] Amanda Ripley writes, "The United States routinely spends more tax dollars per high-school athlete than per high-school math student—unlike most countries worldwide. And we wonder why we lag in international education rankings."

Are sports important? Of course they are, in their appropriate place. Are they more important than math? English? Social studies? No, no, and no, unless, of course, you are that rare breed, the "one and done" basketball prodigy who miraculously graduates from high school, attends a major Division I university (classes optional), and moves on to the pros without anyone ever checking his GPA.

Of course, sports at the scholastic level can also provide fantastic opportunities to experience hard work, physical enrichment, and the tricky dynamics of teamwork as well as character-building lessons in humility, hard work, and failure. These are all very important aspects of child development that can be missed if children are confined to the classroom. But do they need to be strictly organized, with many of them at intense and highly competitive levels?

Athletics are deeply woven into the fabric of America's educational system, especially in middle and upper schools. International exchange students agree that American kids seem to pay as much or more attention to sports than they do to academics.

Igarashi, a sixteen-year-old boy from Osaka, Japan, was amazed when he arrived in Alabama and attended his first day of school. Everyone asked him if he liked football, but no one asked him if he liked math or science. Igarashi saw hundreds of kids in the halls and classrooms wearing football jerseys and T-shirts, and he felt out of place in his Einstein T-shirt, especially when so many students kept asking him who the guy on his shirt was supposed to be.

Back in Osaka, Igarashi enjoyed playing soccer, but when he did have time to play in between classes and studying, it was usually in an empty parking lot near his school. None of his friends played organized sports, unless they attended a special camp during the summer.

By the time American kids reach eighth grade, they spend more than twice the time that Japanese or Korean kids do participating in sports. According to *The Atlantic's* Amanda Ripley, a 2010 study published in the *Journal of Advanced Academics* said that in countries such as Finland and Germany with more-holistic, less hard-driving education systems than those predominant in Asia, many kids play club sports in their local towns—outside of school.[11]

Most schools in Europe and Asia do not organize age-specific teams with coaches, transportation, and insurance, unlike in America, where sports are glorified, often to a point where students must deal with unreasonable expectations spurred on by peers, teachers, coaches—and parents.

In 1961, the sociologist James Coleman observed that a visitor entering an American high school would most likely first encounter a trophy case, and that most, if not all of the trophies would be for winning a sporting event, not a scholastic victory. Coleman suggested that the guest would think that he was entering an athletic club instead of a school.

Friday Night Lights to the Rescue

How did we come to this? As priorities have changed, more and more students are heading out for the practice field in lieu of spending extra time in the classroom. For example, in 2012 at Shawnee High School in New Jersey, with largely white students from middle- and upper-income homes, "only 17 percent of the school's juniors and seniors took at least one Advanced Placement test, but 50 percent of the eleventh- and twelfth-grade students at the school were involved in school sports."[12]

How has the sandlot, pickup ball of yesteryear evolved into today's high-tech, high-stakes world of scholastic sports, just a stone's throw from the booster-fueled, winner-take-all atmosphere of collegiate athletic departments and televised NCAA games that financially benefit the schools but not necessarily the students?

It all began in Texas, home of the classic television program *Friday Night Lights*. On a fall day in Dallas in November 1898, the Wall School of Honey Grove played St. Matthew's Grammar School of Dallas in football, winning 5–0.[13] This historic event was, according to Texas historians, the first recorded football game between two high school teams in their state. It wasn't long before organized sports took over, replacing in many neighborhoods the random pickup games that were a longtime staple for children of all ages. Eventually, schools took over the organizing and management of these activities, hoping to keep the children from cheating too much and knocking each other's brains in. This trend started in elite private schools and gradually became the norm in public schools across the country. New York City inaugurated its own Public Schools Athletic League in 1903, staging a track-and-field event for over a thousand boys at Madison Square Garden during the Christmas holidays.

Educators thought that sports would preserve and enhance masculinity among boys as well as keeping them from bad behavior, like running with the wrong crowd or doing anything illegal.

As Amanda Ripley explains, "'Muscular Christianity,'" fashionable during the Victorian era, prescribed sports as a sort of moral vaccine against the tumult of rapid economic growth. 'In life, as in a foot-ball game,' Theodore Roosevelt wrote in an essay on "The American Boy" in 1900, 'the principle to follow is: Hit the line hard; don't foul and don't shirk, but hit the line hard!'"[14]

Basketball, created in 1892 by James Naismith, caught on quickly, largely because it could be played indoors and did not encourage violent play.

With athletic fields and gymnasiums being built in more and more communities, organized sports became a centerpiece for many towns, villages and cities. Organized youth sports created a stimulating culture to go along with them, including hyper-competitive children, overzealous parents and coaches, some of whom are currently earning more money than everyday classroom teachers.

Critics of these developments continue to wonder aloud whether our tax dollars ought to be spent this way. Some of these sports, especially American football, have proven to pose great risk to our childrens' health, specifically through concussions and other serious injuries.

The trend to add more sports to the high school menu is being bucked more and more recently, often successfully, in football-crazed states throughout the country, where a concerted effort is going on to prioritize academic success over filling school trophy cases with more athletic victories. For some communities, this decision has been made because of a need to cut costs (equipping a football team is a very expensive undertaking), as well as the pressure to provide equal funding for female athletes and their teams.

But with the Bush and Obama administrations pushing new, more stringent federal guidelines that tie student and school performance to teacher pay and state and federal funding, more and more school districts are putting on a full-court press to raise their scores and increase graduation rates to keep the dollars flowing from state and federal coffers. And, of course, some schools are getting it right just because it's the best thing for their kids. Hopefully, we have gotten past the point in the 1980s when Dexter Manley, an All-Pro linebacker in the National Football League, publicly stated that because of his success on the football field, he had been continually promoted and then graduated through both his high school and college career in spite of the fact that he could barely read.[15]

Not Everyone Can Play Quarterback

Sports provide a good example for the dilemma that parents face in our competitive society. What should a parent's role be in all of this? Shall we each grab our athletically inclined children and push them onto the field to take advantage of all that competitive team sports offer, or lock them in their rooms at home to protect them from the vagaries of those very same experiences? What's a parent to do? And what about those parents whose children will never play quarterback or serve as captain of the basketball team?

Sports can be intimidating and stressful for children, especially when they feel pressured to win. And if children focus too much on winning and losing—usually cajoled either way by an adult—they may question their self-worth, especially when they feel disappointment from their coaches and parents.

It is important for your children to understand that their self-worth is not based on whether they win or lose the game or whether they play a starring role in that outcome.[16] Children should participate in athletics because they *want* to, not because their parents push them into doing it. Children should also understand that the goal of sports is to learn from your mistakes and reach your full potential as a player and a teammate. There will be ups and downs in any sport, as there are in life, but the effort that your children put into the game and take away from it is what will stick with them forever.[17]

It's not just a question of whether your child will excel. There are roles for bench players in almost every sport, and the experience of riding the pine can be valuable. The challenge for any parent is to yield, allowing the child to decide how much of a student athlete he or she wants to be. Otherwise, this will lead to apathy about participating and/or making his or her best effort or a feeling of being overwhelmed, which often leads to anxiety, disruptive behavior, poor attendance at games, and, ultimately, burnout.

The best we can do as parents is to guide our children to balance what's in their heads with what is moving in their feet. We can play a significant role in helping our kids make the most of both academics and athletics, but ultimately the choices have to rest with them. As they get older, they come to understand the consequences of their choices. Our job is merely to point out these consequences and then support their passions. It is important to remember that sports are games and are supposed to be fun. The critical issue is that children feel good about themselves. That doesn't mean that they should not work hard, train hard, and be involved; it's just that when they are badgered to perform at a level that they don't want to or can't sustain, some kids can be left with self-image and self-esteem issues. Others end up quitting or burning out early, effectively rendering what started out as something fun to do into something full of frustration and disappointment for those around them. This can leave children with a pronounced sense of failure, of not having followed through on something that they originally liked and in which they had some ability to do well. The fallout from any of these scenarios can last well into adulthood.

CHAPTER 5: HOW OVERPARENTING
AFFECTS YOUR CHILD—AND YOU

With parents today feeling increased pressure to launch their children into the world with all the tools and advantages needed to be successful, we must examine the adverse effects of this behavior for children and parents alike. Even though the media may sensationalize the issue with headlines such as "From China to France to America: A Backlash against Overprotective Parents"[1] or "Overprotective Parenting: A Growing Worldwide Problem"[2] or "Children with Controlling 'Helicopter Parents' More Likely to Be Depressed,"[3] these troubling notices do not appear out of thin air or without reason, and they should be a subject of our concern.

This is because the effects of overparenting go far beyond teenage children's complaining about their parents' nagging them and enforcing what seem to the children to be unreasonable curfews or limits on where they can go in the neighborhood and with whom. In fact, the effects of overparenting begin much earlier than most people think. From the first time a mother pampers her child when she barely scrapes her knee to the phone calls that a father makes to try to secure a spot for his kid in a Wall Street firm—and all the interventions in between—well-meaning parents run the risk of creating a falsely entitled, overly coddled, and dependent child, one long on laziness and short on self-esteem, lost without someone's intervening on her behalf to take care of whatever problem she may be facing. These children may suffer from compromised creativity, have difficulty making their own choices, encounter trouble in dealing with failure, have problems with bouncing back from setbacks, and lack the ability to select or do things entirely on their own—at any age. Overparenting can reinforce a tendency in children to blame others for their own shortcomings, and the ones they ultimately blame are their parents. To make matters worse, these character traits and the inability to deal successfully with life's issues continue to follow these children well into adulthood. Many of them will be unable to actually maximize their potential or fully take care of themselves without the urge to constantly look for a parent, life coach, or some other type of counselor to guide or rescue them.

Intensive Parenting

At the core of overparenting lies the psychological roots for why it happens. Why the push to try so hard? What makes parents so intense? Why do so many perceive their children, irrespective of their age, as vulnerable and incapable, if not helpless? What has prompted this mad rush to constantly monitor and protect our children? While some of the reasons have been explored in Chapter 3, it is worth reexamining some of the underlying roots of why parents are driven to behave like this.

It used to be the job of parents to expose their kids to the outside world by simply throwing them into the metaphorical pool of life and hoping that they could swim or by managing the amount of external input that they received, dosing out "the real world" a little at a time. But many parents today seem hell-bent on protecting their children from what they consider to be the perils of the outside world, which, if you are an overly protective parent, can be almost anything. More and more research suggests that this type of overly intensive parenting can be harmful for children and, not coincidentally, not very good for you as their parent. No matter what type of parent you might be, if you do not allow your child to make mistakes, learn coping skills, develop independence, and ultimately become self-sufficient, you simply have not done your job. Parenting is not about merely raising children by planning and trying to engineer a successful outcome for them. Your job as a parent is to help transition, if not slingshot, a whole, developing young adult—with his or her very own personality—into the world.

When parents are too intense, their children often fail to develop skills that they will need throughout their life. These include time management, strategizing, prioritizing, and the ins and outs of negotiating. It begins when you first feed your child and continues with his or her first tussle at home with a sibling or with another kid in nursery school or on the playground. Children subjected to too much overparenting are prone to demonstrate less spontaneity, enjoyment, and initiative when it comes to how they spend their leisure time. Children raised by intensive parents also lean toward becoming less attentive to the feelings of others. This lack of empathy may be a result of constantly looking over their shoulders to see how they are doing in the eyes of the one person they think matters: their parent. This approach to life is clearly very limiting for children, and they may never get to successfully decide what they themselves want to do or learn how to internalize and appreciate how good of a job they have done.

When these kids finally do leave home, at whatever age, they do so with a continuous need to check on how they are doing in their parents' eyes, as if they are always looking over their shoulders to get approval or validation. Their parents, who have somewhat crippled their children in the process of raising them, also seem to want to keep that umbilical cord intact. This leads to a bilateral and ongoing effort to continue access to the parents via email, texting, and phone. The habits developed through late childhood and early adolescence continue holding the children back from becoming their own people as they get older. They become essentially infantile and insecure, trapped in a constant state of uncertainty and dependency, as if they are always asking for permission or approval because they are terrified of jumping ahead on their own. At the same time, they have an ongoing fantasy that has been perpetuated by this interaction: that should there be a problem, there will never really be any major consequences for them, and their parents or someone else will always be there to jump in and fix the issue or bail them out of difficult situations. It should be no surprise when many overparented kids make poor choices, flounder, blame others, and then attempt to cope by using alcohol and an assortment of drugs as well as by resorting to a series of sexual relationships. By that time, though, they unfortunately discover that their parents cannot always bail them out, make it right, or protect them from the consequences of their behavior, and they do not have the interpersonal resources to do it on their own.

The Overparenting Equation:
Cause and Effect for Your Child and You

Actions have consequences. But in today's world, where the stakes seem much higher and our lives are coming under unprecedented scrutiny, it's becoming more and more difficult as parents to feel confident in our choices. While we can't always predict the consequences of those choices, we must always deal with how they affect our children and us.

Times have changed. In previous generations, parents who "let their kids run wild" were viewed with disdain by neighbors, but subjected to no greater sanction than head wagging and disapproving gossip in the community. Today, such situations are far more likely to result in a call to Child Protective Services, with subsequent legal intervention and the threat of losing custody of your child.

"We raised our three children without any television and with a very limited amount of computer time," says Jamie, from Columbia, South Carolina. "They played outdoors a lot with no adult supervised sports until they played baseball and basketball in middle school. It was very lonely unless we had playdates. We lived in a low-income neighborhood so I could stay home with them and make this happen. I would've had to work full-time for us to live in a better neighborhood. Our neighbors thought we were crazy. But as kids grow, it's practically impossible to find places where they can play freely without an adult accusing you of neglect."

So, we keep asking ourselves, when it comes to our own flesh and blood, our beloved children, are we doing too much or too little? Can my kid make it if I'm poor? Isn't having plenty of money the ticket to a perfect future?

"I teach in a very diverse community with children of drug addicts and ex-cons and kids whose parents are very well educated and successful," says Larry, a middle school teacher in Phoenix, Arizona. "There is a big range of socioeconomic levels, and in terms of classroom behavior, the low socioeconomic students are starting to outshine the high socioeconomic ones. I think it's because outside of school the 'better-off' students never get a break from their nonstop schedule of practices, lessons, and playdates, leaving them with very little time for self-directed play. The supposedly 'lesser off' kids may have quite a few hassles at home and in their neighborhoods, and as a result they learn a lot more about dealing with things and negotiating their way through it all."

Overparenting can send a variety of messages to your children. Most, if not all of these messages, are better not sent at all. The rule of cause and effect essentially goes like this: for every parental action, there is a child's reaction, for better or for worse, with a lot of reality in between. Your concern should not be about any one singular incident and how you respond to it, unless something very traumatic has occurred. In that case, you should probably seek outside help for your family. Generally, though, you should be deeply concerned about any patterns of overparenting you notice yourself becoming comfortable with and repeating. While your behavior may seem to be habitual, which can deceptively give the feeling that it is OK, these questionable patterns can have very negative effects on your children—and you. They can put you in a mode where you are not looking at every situation independently and instead you are treating your children as if they are always the same and not constantly changing, as most children do. In fact, not looking at every situation independently can cause a parent to begin to stereotype or scapegoat a child as "the smart one" or the "oppositional one." It's no joke that as soon as we figure out what phase our kids are in and how to deal with it, they are on to the next one! This means that any stereotypical reaction you may employ to react to their behavior, such as "you're lazy," will fast become a losing proposition for them and you. With these principles in mind, it would be wise to take a deeper look at the overparenting equation, that is, what happens when you make certain choices and the consequences they create—for your children and you. It is important to also recognize that all children are different, even those with the same parents, so you really need to think through what each child is like, what works for each one, and what you need to tailor to each one's distinctive personality and circumstances, and when some of what the child does changes, you need to change your perception and response as well.

In order to understand the risks and results of overparenting, we would do well to reexamine the parental archetypes that we presented in Chapter 1, which demonstrate much of this behavior. Each personality presents specific risks, which may trigger a variety of results, for parents as well as children. See if you can identify yourself among these archetypes and whether you recognize the risks and results. Within each archetypal grouping, we will discuss the overall weight of these risks and results. While the short-term effects may not be so bad, the long-term consequences are not encouraging or to be taken lightly. It is worth pointing out again that at times of crisis we all may slide into one or more of these roles, which is quite understandable. It becomes problematic, however, if you remain stuck there or include your child in your counterproductive behavior.

GUARDIAN ANGELS
The Protector
Risk: These parents will do almost anything to protect their child.
Result for Child: The child never learns to take chances or risk failure.
Result for Parents: The parents must work harder to support the appropriate development of the child's independence.
The Hyper-Protector
Risk: These parents keep their child from participating in normal activities.
Result for Child: The child feels left out and becomes alienated.
Result for Parents: The parents need to spend more time helping the child become social.

The Intervener

Risk: These parents put their nose in the child's business against her will.

Result for Child: The child can't solve problems on her own.

Result for Parents: The parents must figure out how to empower the child to solve problems on her own.

The Anxiety Maker

Risk: These parents openly worry about everything concerning their child.

Result for Child: The child grows up anxious about everything.

Result for Parents: The parents must deal with the child's increased anxiety levels.

Overparenting = A Lack of Trust

Overprotective parents unintentionally send out a message to their children that they are incapable of handling things by themselves, and need their parent's input to make sure that they "get it right." For children, that simply translates into a feeling that their parents do not trust them, which is true, no matter what the parents may say. When parents step in to take over even the most basic transactions that a child is capable of doing for himself, the message is that they do not trust their child to manage even the minor ups and downs of life. This means that, ultimately, the parents don't make things easier for their child, but rather inhibit the child's growth and, in the process of jumping in, give their child permission to be lazy, be unmotivated, and believe that he is not responsible for his actions, and leave the child with feelings of inadequacy and a lack of confidence.

Overparenting also contributes to other kinds of trust issues in children. If parents do not trust what is happening in the world, and consistently transmit their own fears about the world to their children, those kids will also grow up suspecting everything around them. That again leads to a sense that the world is more dangerous than it is, that nothing can be trusted, and that there may be real danger lurking around any corner. This is not the legacy that most parents want to leave their children, when they are just trying to help them out.

Overparenting = Inadequate Life Skills

When parents intervene, or have the maids and nannies do so for their children, to ensure that they do not have to be burdened with any of life's mundane tasks, such as learning to tie their shoelaces, dry themselves, comb their own hair, or pick up after themselves, they are certainly not helping their children grow up and accept responsibility for themselves. In fact, they are doing quite the opposite, in relaying the message that those tasks are unimportant, and someone else will do them, so that their children can just do the important things, such as being brilliant at building with wooden blocks or LEGO.

Luanne, an elementary school teacher, told a story about going on an overnight school trip with fifth- and sixth-graders where she discovered that many of the kids had never learned to get dressed by themselves, make their own beds, or set the table for a meal. Luanne was flummoxed. What other basic life skills might these kids be lacking, she wondered, and how will that bode for their future in middle and secondary school? She thought that maybe her classroom curriculum should be expanded to include these things, because they obviously weren't being taught at home.

Are these kids victims of overparenting, *under*parenting, or neglect?

Judy, a longtime acquaintance, grew up in New York City during the 1940s and 1950s, and while her family was not wealthy, per se,

Judy had a nanny who looked after her and kept the house in order. This arrangement was in place until Judy went to college. Well, a few weeks after she arrived, she had quite a shock when she went to get dressed one morning and realized that she had no clean underwear. In fact, when she began looking in earnest, she realized that for the past three weeks, she had been discarding her worn clothes randomly around her room, without a single thought of putting them in a hamper or cleaning them. Laundry? What's that? Judy's nanny had always picked up her clothes and made sure they were all washed, ironed, folded, and made ready for Judy's next wearing. So, Judy's first major learning curve in college should have been doing her own laundry. But in Judy's case, and we suspect that it could be the same with many others, she simply went shopping that day for new underwear and hired another student to do her laundry. Apparently, this habit hasn't gone out of style, and many students today are heading off to college without a clue about how to take care of basic things for themselves. Some colleges have prepared for this and provide weekly laundry services.

While there have been no studies that we know of to find out how many children over the age of eighteen know how to change a light bulb, we can probably go out on a limb and guess that the number is shockingly low. Will those kids learn any fundamental life skills such as that during their college years? Probably not. So, what favors are parents doing their children when they spare them the "burden" of learning how to take care of themselves while they are growing up? A child who grows up like this will certainly tax his or her spouse, who may feel like he or she has taken the role of the maid, nanny, or parent in picking up after her spouse, unless they are sufficiently wealthy that they can afford a nanny or a maid from day one.

TYPE As

The Overachiever

Risk: These parents set unreachable expectations.

Result for Child: The child feels as if he can never satisfy anyone.

Result for Parents: The parents may regret the extra pressure placed on the child.

The Controller

Risk: These parents insist on making choices for their child.

Result for Child: The child can't think for himself.

Result for Parents: The parents must take extra time to deal with a needy child.

The Negotiator

Risk: These parents do not allow their child to deal with difficult situations alone.

Result for Child: The child's ability to fend for himself is compromised.

Result for Parents: The parents will not relax and trust their child's ability to cope.

The Micromanager

Risk: These parents take drastic measures to control the outcomes of the child's life.

Result for Child: The child fears making mistakes and loses learning moments.

Result for Parents: The parents lose the chance to see their child learn from mistakes.

Overparenting = Fear of Failure

Fear of failure often occurs when parents who are already overinvolved with their kids reward them for every little activity or action.

It is almost as if every breath they take becomes a major event, like with your first child, and in turn those children often develop a false sense of accomplishment and specialness.

According to Katherine Ozment in *Boston Magazine*, Carol Dweck, the author of *Mindset: The New Psychology of Success*, feels that too much praise can be counterproductive. Dweck says that "when we tell kids that they are gifted, rather than hardworking, they can develop a fear of failing that leads to an unwillingness to take the risks necessary for true learning." We see evidence of that among children in gifted and talented programs who become stressed out trying to keep up with the expectations placed on them by teachers—and parents.

"Kids who are told that they're hard workers, in contrast, are more willing to take on challenges and better able to bounce back from mistakes," Dreck told Ozment. "The psychological community now holds that incessant praise actually works against parents' intentions. You don't gain self-esteem first, then achieve great things. You work hard, fail, pick yourself up, try again, accomplish something new, and *then* feel pretty good about yourself."[4]

Magnifying every action and activity our children come up with only sets them up to expect that everyone will make a big fuss over everything they do and/or say. That leads to disappointment in the real world, few problem-solving skills, a lack of perseverance, and failure when hardships do occur. When problems arise, which happens to *everybody*, they don't know what to do and have a tantrum or just plain fold. When a child is young, this can be corrected with extra effort by parents, peers, and teachers to deal with their fragile emotions and bolster their self-confidence, while trying to help them learn to manage problems themselves. When they grow older, it is often too late for them to learn how to take care of issues, let alone push forward with any real tenacity.

Overparenting = Reduced Self-Esteem

As Steve Baskin discusses in *Psychology Today*, when author Nathaniel Branden published *The Psychology of Self-Esteem* in 1969, he reconfigured how we consider psychoanalysis and the ways in which we look at ourselves. Branden's groundbreaking philosophy was radically different than the status quo of that era and asked people to reexamine their very nature as humans.

The Psychology of Self-Esteem redefined the relationship of reason to emotion, Baskin explains, including the nature of free will, and the powerful impact of self esteem on motivation, work, friendship, sex, and romantic love.[5]

According to Dr. Branden, "self-esteem is an essential human need that is vital for survival and normal, healthy development. It arises automatically from within, based on a person's beliefs and consciousness and occurs in conjunction with a person's thoughts, behaviors, feelings, and actions."[6]

Branden's book prompted parents to begin doing whatever they thought was necessary to boost their children's self-esteem. We call it "parenting on steroids" because it led to a lot of artificial "pumping up" of children's egos, all in an effort to boost their self-esteem and self-worth. How else do you explain kids on losing sports teams receiving trophies simply for participating or students bringing home lackluster grades, only to be stroked and told that they must have done their best and that they should feel good about themselves? That sort of recognition and empty praise has proved to produce poor performance, acceptance of mediocrity, and unhealthy personality traits in children as they develop.

For example, a landmark 2007 study from Columbia University found that kids who are continually told that they are smart tend to avoid activities where they don't excel, essentially selling themselves short for fear of failure.[7]

This kind of coddling to promote self-esteem, which often comes with an acceptance of mediocre performance, may explain record-high rates of narcissism among today's young adults.[8] We see evidence of that in almost every classroom, including private, public, and parochial schools.

Indulging our children with bloated praise and meaningless trophies will not go very far toward supporting successful, satisfied kids. Learning how to fail and bravely move forward is part of growing up—for everyone. Self-esteem is an essential human need that is vital for survival and normal, healthy development. It should begin at a young age.

As psychologist Abraham Maslow explained in his work on the human hierarchy of needs, self-esteem is one of the basic human motivations. Maslow suggested that people need esteem from other people as well as from their own self-respect. Both of these needs must be fulfilled in order for an individual to grow as a person and achieve self-actualization.

The issue is not artificially trying to pump our children up to make them feel good and bolster their self-esteem. It is helping them learn to master situations so that they can feel good about and respect themselves for what they have accomplished. This will also prevent them from seeking out other children who are also struggling with low self-esteem, who accept and then validate each other's poor performance. This is particularly an issue among teenagers, who tend to bond together and support each other's bad behavior. As parents, we play a central role in the development of our children's self-esteem, and it is critical to examine what we can realistically do in this regard to ensure that our children develop properly.

BUDDIES

The Best-Friender

Risk: These parents constantly crave the companionship of their child.
Result for Child: The child has little life of her own and becomes a puppet of her parent.
Result for Parents: The parents have no life of their own, and when the child eventually leaves, they are crushed.

The Assister

Risk: These parents help the child, even when she doesn't need it.
Result for Child: The child never learns to be self-sufficient.
Result for Parents: The parents don't really take care of their own needs.

The Spoiler

Risk: These parents will do anything to indulge their child.
Result for Child: The child expects anything that he wants to be provided.
Result for Parents: The parents lose their own sense of working for something.

The Smotherer

Risk: These parents overwhelm the child with too much attention.
Result for Child: The child can't develop a sense of his own independence.
Result for Parents: The parents sacrifice their own independence.

Overparenting = Feelings of Entitlement

Many parents are so overprotective of their children that the children do not learn to take responsibility, accept the natural consequence of their actions, and learn from their mistakes. This notion that they can do whatever they want, that the rules don't apply to them, and that if a problem develops, their parents will jump in and help, provides a sense that they are really not responsible or accountable for anything and, therefore, they do not learn from their actions. This well-meaning but needless protection may cause these children to develop a sense of entitlement that will end up crippling their development while creating problems for them as they interact with others. Parents who feel entitled themselves, be it from their own success or being born into the right family, may find it difficult to work with their child's school in a trusting, cooperative, and positive manner, which only tends to impede their child's progress in school. The result is that the staff at the school are often resentful, and at some point distance themselves from the child, who they will just see as spoiled.

Entitlement then becomes a tricky issue to deal with, rather like bad karma. Just as the world has its own way of filtering out injustice and balancing the scales of who gets what they deserve, what goes around may come back to haunt you, or, in the case of overly entitled kids becoming overly entitled adults, it may come back to haunt them and their own children.

Overparenting = Lack of Creativity

Peter Gray, an evolutionary psychologist at Boston College, who edited the spring 2011 issue of the *American Journal of Play*, explains that free, unstructured play helps children learn how to get along with others, control their emotions, and develop their imaginations.[9] Does this sound like the pool of children from which you want your kid to be selecting for his or her playdates?

How could it have happened that kids and play are no longer guaranteed to be entirely synonymous? Since the 1950s, Gray says, there's been a steady decline in the time American children spend playing on their own.

A study by the University of Maryland's Sandra Hofferth found that, between 1981 and 1997, American kids ages six to eight spent 25 percent less time engaged in free play, while their classroom time rose by 18 percent. Meanwhile, their homework time increased by 145 percent, and the time they spent shopping with their parents rose by 168 percent. When Hofferth updated her research in 2003, free time continued to decline, while study time increased another 32 percent.[10] Who knows what happened to shopping time, but if the amount of goods that kids seem to have today is any indication, it has not declined at all.

Family psychologists point out that during the past twenty-five years the value of free time in childhood has been largely forgotten. But all the hours and money spent honing artistic, athletic, and academic skills can actually tamp down on children's creativity, because kids aren't left with any spare moments to read, draw, or imagine on their own.[11]

By overscheduling children's lives, parents inadvertently prohibit them from developing the creative skill sets that foster problem solving, resiliency and self-confidence down the road. Free, unstructured time, when children can daydream, fantasize, and look at their lives and work out solutions to what they see as life's problems, allows creativity to develop. When people are too busy, they don't have the time or the mental space to be able to do that.

The iconic psychoanalyst Bruno Bettelheim explains that a child's inner world becomes impoverished without sufficient mental room for play. "Play is the work of the child,"[12] he said, a central mechanism through which children get acquainted with the surrounding world and develop a sense of independence and separation. Intensive parenting, which is built on intense, hands-on supervision, significantly limits play and puts our children at risk.

PRODUCERS

The Consumer
Risk: These parents put a price tag on everything concerning their child.
Result for Child: The child considers herself to be unrealistically special, and believes that school is just for academic performance and not social skill development.
Result for Parents: The parents alienate people around them.

The Blamer
Risk: These parents put blame on others instead of facing consequences.
Result for Child: The child feels entitled to behave however he chooses, because it's not his fault.
Result for Parents: The parents alienate people around them.

The Delegator
Risk: These parents view their child as a project.
Result for Child: The child is not sure who loves him or is responsible for him.
Result for Parents: The parents lose their chance to really know their child.

The Disrespecter
Risk: These parents act out their superiority complex on adults responsible for their child.

Result for Child: The parents undermine and essentially disrespect their child.

Result for Parents: The parents alienate people around them.

Overparenting = Irresponsible and Unaccountable Young Adults

Why is it that when children screw up or don't achieve what they want, more and more parents seem so willing to blame someone else instead of holding their own child—and themselves in some cases—accountable?

If your child cheats on a test, do you blame the teacher because the test is too hard? Do you blame your child's eye doctor because he forgot to tell you that your kid has a "wandering eye"? Or do you blame the government for insisting on all these tests in the first place? Some of those excuses will stick, won't they? If you keep looking to excuse your child from being accountable for his actions, you are helping him also accept the idea that he is not accountable for what happened, and teaching him to behave in the same way as you have. Your kid will become as arrogant and irresponsible as you have been when you try to blame someone else for your child's shortcomings. The idea of blaming someone else means that you don't have to accept responsibility for what happened, and you then don't have to make an effort to make things better.

Fortunately, the fact that some things in this complex world in which we live are cut and dry and right or wrong is not hard to establish. Cheating is wrong, no matter how you slice it, and it appears in many forms. Some of them are not so easy to referee, and when it comes to crime and punishment, figuring out what punishment is proportional to the crime is even more difficult. How you determine what a proper reaction or consequence might be as opposed to just overreacting can be quite tricky, but ignoring the issue or blaming someone else for it is never an answer. Determining right and wrong and what the consequences should be depends on your own moral code as a parent, but it is a subject you can discuss with other parents or staff at school. For some people, trying to determine this is very difficult, and it only gets harder when you are trying to get a leg up on everyone else on behalf of your child.

Overparenting = Bad Role Modeling

Crissy and Lauren are in an afterschool program at their middle school in a suburb of Minneapolis, Minnesota. One day, while they were messing around in the library, making videos on their phones, Crissy hit Lauren in the mouth by accident and busted up her lip pretty badly. It was a total accident. They went to the nurse right away, who called Lauren's mother, who came immediately (as if she had been waiting outside the school for such an occasion) and took her daughter to the local emergency room, where she got a few stitches. As soon as Lauren and her mother got home, Lauren called Crissy to give her the lowdown on her stitches and the cute guy working as a nurse in the ER, while Lauren's mother emailed the school, complaining bitterly about its lack of proper supervision. She then called Crissy's house to report the incident to her parents, accusing Crissy of hitting her daughter intentionally. She kept demanding an apology, even when Lauren insisted that it had been a total accident.

Lauren's mother, triggered by an irrational need to intervene on behalf of her child, is a good example of what overparenting can look like. What we say to our children is important, of course, but our actions play a bigger role in modeling positive and realistic behavior. The sad part of this story is that the kids were ready to move on with their friendship until the parents got involved and made it worse.

Overparenting = Inept Children

As our children develop, we must allow them the chance to take responsibility for some basics in life, such as buttering their own toast, picking up their own clothes, putting away their toys when they finish playing with them, and helping with setting or clearing the dining room table. Not allowing children to do any form of chores or assume any responsibility because they may not get it right or because there is a maid who will do these things for them is not doing them a favor. Children must be encouraged to take responsibility at home as they are growing up, so that by the time they become teenagers they are somewhat self-reliant, especially when it comes to life's basic needs. If they do not learn this before they leave home, they will never know how to manage on their own when they leave home, whether that means attending college, taking a job away from home, or enlisting in the armed forces. Learning to do things for themselves is also a way in which children learn to build self-esteem, take pride and responsibility in the commitments they make, and in turn feel good about themselves. Not letting them learn to do this essentially deprives them of learning how to move forward by themselves when you or someone else is not around.

Learning to do chores, even if they are not done perfectly by a six-year-old, allows you and your child to accept that he or she may not always do it perfectly. Dishes do break, even when a parent does them at times, and children can accept that no one, including their parents, is perfect, and they make mistakes, but at least they are trying to do things and help out.

This process also helps your children when you have realistic, age-appropriate expectations for them and helps them appreciate that if it doesn't work out quite right all the time, it is not the end of the world.

If this doesn't happen, by the time children are sixteen or seventeen years old, they will feel incapable of doing *anything* right or meeting any of your expectations.

Coddling is not a recipe for success. Spoiling your children is harmful. It does not empower them to make confident decisions. For example, when it comes time for high school seniors to make decisions about where they want to apply to college, they have to use at least some of their own judgment and learn to work with someone who is more knowledgeable in that area, such as their school counselor. If they end up at a college that's not right for them, it is not the end of the world. It happens all the time and can be fixed. It's a learning opportunity for children, not a chance for you to bemoan their choices or for them to complain forever that it was your fault that they didn't do well, that they didn't like the place they went to, or that they sabotaged themselves because they didn't feel like they participated in the decision.

ACCESSORIES

The Cheerleader
Risk: These parents think their children are the "best" at everything they do.
Result for Child: The child develops a false sense of accomplishment.
Result for Parents: The parents perpetuate a false sense of reality.

The Carpooler
Risk: These parents can't stop gossiping about their child's teachers and school.
Result for Child: The child is humiliated by the parents' loose lips.
Result for Parents: The parents alienate people around them.

The Trophy Giver

Risk: These parents want their child to be a "winner" at everything he or she does.

Result for Child: The child grows up without a realistic view of the world.

Result for Parents: The parents lessen the value of their own achievements.

The Maturity Killer

Risk: These parents always treat their child like a "child."

Result for Child: The child's psychological and emotional growth is stunted.

Result for Parents: The parents miss out on the evolving parent-child relationship.

Overparenting = Increased Anxiety

When we become too emotionally involved in the issues facing our children, we ramp up the stakes unreasonably high and create way too much pressure for our kids. Children by nature want to please their parents, but when their anxiety to do so is very high, they have little room to live their lives and balance out what they want as well. The fallout from this can be far-reaching.

A study by Columbia University psychology professor Suniya Luthar reveals that pushing kids can be just as bad for them as attending to their every desire. Luthar found that the children of upper-class, highly educated parents in the Northeast are increasingly anxious and depressed. Children with "high perfectionist strivings" were likely to see achievement failures as personal failures. Luthar also found that "being constantly shuttled between activities—spending all that time in the SUV with Mom or Dad—ends up leaving suburban adolescents feeling *more* isolated from their parents."[13] We suspect that their parents also feel more isolated from them as well, as they get to feel like chauffeurs and not like parents.

According to the Anxiety and Depression Association of America, anxiety disorders affect one in eight children. Research shows that children with untreated anxiety disorders are at higher risk of performing poorly in school, missing out on important social experiences, and engaging in substance abuse. Anxiety disorders also occur with other disorders, such as depression, eating disorders, and attention-deficit/hyperactivity disorder (ADHD). With treatment and support, your child can learn how to successfully manage the symptoms of an anxiety disorder and live a normal childhood.[14]

With "normal," good parenting, however, anxiety disorders may not develop in the first place. In fact, our children's anxiety can often remain at normal levels when parents take a step back, relax, and let life happen. We should all take notice that an overanxious parent who constantly magnifies issues can escalate a child's anxiety levels, sometimes to the point where he or she will become terrified of everything.

Overparenting = Compromised Resilience

When parents try to overprotect or coddle their children, they are providing them with short-term protection at the expense of long-term life skills. By overprotecting children from an unpleasant occurrence, of which life is full, parents are keeping them from learning how to deal with those types of events, or, in essence, to become resilient. A lack of resilience also results from your occasional, small, and simple indulgences. When your son has a little cold and wants to stay home from school, rather than push him to go when you know that he is not very sick, you may want to be the "perfect" parent. This is an excuse to pamper your kid so that you keep him home, where he ends up playing all day, happy to have your constant attention. This can quickly become an indulgence that repeats itself over and over. That may not sound like a bad thing at first, but what are you really teaching your son by indulging these whims? The message you give is that every little sniffle or pain needs special attention and treatment and that school, and ultimately work, can be put off for any sort of minor reason. This approach does not help a child develop maturity and responsibility, and, besides, you might be missing the real reason why he wants to stay home. Could he be having any issues at school? Is he struggling? Being bullied? Being a bully himself? In between hugs, you might want to check out those things.

Children—like all of us—are not always ready to deal with many life events and will hide behind a cold or headache to keep from doing so. Naturally, parents do not want to upset their children, believing that they should not have to deal with unpleasant situations—or at least not too soon. This inclination to protect our children, as noble as it may first appear, does not give them a chance to learn how to cope with whatever it is they need to wrestle with, be it loud teachers, teasing, not getting what they want, or wishing that they could just stay home and watch TV. We all know adults who use these same ploys to basically avoid unpleasant circumstances or get what they want. Let your parental resolve and resilience teach your children how to develop theirs. You are their role models, and "do as I do, not just as I say" is the more accurate mantra.

Does Overparenting Affect You, Too?

It surely does! We can see from this list that parents are affected just as much as children by their own overparenting, and in some ways, the long-term consequences for the parent may be worse.

As an adult, you need to create a life of your own, and your self-esteem and self-worth should be driven by your own successes, activities and relationships—not just those of your children. It's all fine and good for you to feel pleased by their accomplishments, but if your life is totally caught up in how your child lives his or hers, you will never be happy. You will always be hanging on to how well—or not—they are living up to your expectations.

There is no way that anyone—your child or your spouse—can fully meet your hopes and expectations all the time. If your levels of self-esteem and self-worth are determined too much by how your child is doing, then you will always be living on the edge of your seat, worrying about how his or her next act will play out. That means that the way in which you value yourself will be contingent upon how well your child performs—compared to your expectations—in his or her own life.

What if they don't do as well as you think they should? Like everyone else, they will have ups and downs, but that roller coaster—just like yours—is about *their* life and goals—not yours. So if you are always trying to manage your child's life, you will never be living your own.

If you have been constantly invested in overseeing or managing your child's life, then you risk becoming not just an empty nester, but also a very depressed, sad and lonely person. You will quickly find that while you may have socialized with the parents of your children's friends, those relationships fade when your kids leave home and you have to invent new ones.

While it may be true, as the saying goes, that you are only as happy as your unhappiest child, you also have to develop other things in your own life, regardless of how and what your child is doing. This becomes even more crucial when they start getting involved with friends in lower school, go out with friends as teenagers or hopefully leave home and go to college.

Why do parents forget so easily that as children—both young and older—we figured out what was going on in the world just as much on our own as we did from our parents? So while it's one thing to explain to a young child that the world is a dangerous place and that they need your protection and input to function or be successful, if you keep that up at the same rate as they grow older, you may get your wish and have a child who fears going out into the world and never leaves home. That means both of you will ultimately have no outside life, and it can create a very unhappy, angry, co-dependent relationship, one in which the child blames the parent for never having a life and the parent continues trying to help the child manage their own life, even into adulthood. Years of clinical experience repeatedly demonstrate that these are some of the most unhappy, unsuccessful people needing help.

Which Child Is Yours?

While it may not be quite so obvious, the subtle effects of overparenting are often regrettable and can be avoided. It would be wise to avoid these pitfalls for yourself, but, most of all, for your innocent children. These parental archetypes often produce a certain type of child whose particular behavior in response to a parent's style can even begin to be recognized during preschool years. While parenting authorities have ascribed catchy names for these children, their behavior is often anything but cute. The biggest challenge we face as parents is to be objective about our own kids before it is too late. When we accomplish that by acknowledging their weaknesses, faults, and strengths, we can also recognize some of our own as well as the choices we make that may push our kids in a direction in which we do not really want them to go. If we are alert, we can nip some of what they do early on in the bud, before they are older and their behavior becomes much more difficult to reverse. Looking beyond the cute nicknames, see if you recognize your child within these groupings.

Teacups: These children are extremely fragile and sensitive about their own discomforts or problems.[15] It is as if they could be easily broken, and they have an extremely difficult time handling criticism or rejection and tend to avoid anything where they might not easily succeed. As these children grow older and encounter challenging high school curricula, college life, and the job market, they tend to stumble and need large doses of external support. As they get older, this often takes the form of subsidies from parents who are guilt-ridden about having raised children with limited coping skills and do not know how to help them move on in any other way.

College counselors see "a rise in digestive and eating disorders, headaches, generalized anxiety disorder, substance abuse, social and school phobias and obsessive-compulsive disorders among students who are perfectionists, and overwork school assignments. Even more alarming is the increase in self-injury—a desperate and poignant cry for relief. Our mental health services can barely keep up with the demand."[16] This shows that these kids cannot extricate themselves from a situation that they have most probably gotten themselves into in the first place, so they create a crisis so that someone, usually a parent, will jump in and bail them out.

Toasties: These kids, who were heavily overloaded from a very young age, have burned out by the time they really need to perform on their own.[17] Their parents overloaded their schedules with performing arts classes, karate, tennis, and tutors. If there was a brochure laying around for something new, these children were surely dragged out the door, into the minivan, across town, and into another "enrichment" program. From a very early age, these kids were so busy in structured settings that they never had sufficient time to relax and just play or hang or do nothing for a while. By the time they hit their middle teenage years, they are often burned out—just when they are becoming aware of the looming pressure to be involved in activities and build a résumé for college. By the time they graduate from high school, they are simply relieved that it's over, and this feeling may last well into their college years and beyond. Without the ongoing supervision and direction they had at home, by the time they get away in college or boarding school, they may lose themselves in "partying." Because they were constantly monitored and never learned how to control and moderate their activities when they were growing up at home, as soon as they are no longer supervised, they lack any direction and often do poorly or get into alcohol and drugs. Many of these kids have no sense of what really interests them or what they care about because they have been directed since early childhood. They may pick a major they don't really care about and then professions that don't really challenge them. In some cases, their lives become a disappointment—to themselves and their parents.

A report from the Harvard Office of Admissions describes some incoming students as "dazed survivors of some bewildering lifelong boot camp."

"Incoming students have been so scheduled, so sleep deprived and pressured, that they come to college too finely tuned," complains one dean of students. "They're like thoroughbreds. If they 'throw a shoe,' they can't recover."[18]

Turtles: As a result of being raised in an atmosphere of privilege, entitlement, and being protected from real-life issues, including those that have affected their parents, these kids assume that everything in their lives will always be fine and that there is no need to hustle or push for anything. They feel that they can just chill and not stress about anything, which often translates into not putting forth the effort to seize opportunities or realize their potential—in the classroom, on the ball field, or in the studio. They skate through life without taking on any challenges that might mess up their hair or make them sweat. This path produces docile, lazy kids who lack general empathy and tend to become apathetic and passionless.[19] This is best illustrated by the old phrase "good things come to those who wait, but the best things come to those who do."

"These kids who come from highly entitled environments, who have been spoiled all their life, have a difficult time in college," says an admissions counselor from an elite liberal arts college in the Northeast. "First of all, they're barely capable of doing their own laundry, and they're clueless when it comes time to sign up for classes and eventually declare a major." Did their parents really do them a favor by paving the way for them?

Tyrants: These kids have grown up with their parents constantly telling them that they are special, that they can do no wrong, and that their poop smells like birthday cake. They feel that they deserve the best of everything, and see no reason why they should not have whatever they want. While they will apply themselves to get what they want and what they feel they are entitled to, if they don't think that they are the center of attention in any given situation, they will let everyone know about it in no uncertain terms.

"I've seen these types gravitate to fraternities," reports one alumnus from a large Midwestern state school. "They were probably a big-shot athlete in high school, and their father was a prominent lawyer or bank executive, so they feel that the world is their oyster. Except at a big university, there are a lot of other big fishes coming from small ponds, and once they get on campus, they find out real quick how insignificant they are. A lot of them can't handle it and end up self-destructing." In truth, these tend to be somewhat narcissistic and entitled kids who not only feel like they deserve whatever they want but resent having to work for it. They think that they can simply take shortcuts or use Mommy's or Daddy's connections to get them where they think they deserve to be.

As a parent, you may recognize some of these traits. Many kids will show traces of some of these characteristics on occasion, and if that's all they do, they will be fine. But before your children grow up and become locked into any of these types, watch out! This behavior is very easy to undo when the child is young—if you recognize it and respond differently to your child—but it is very difficult to undo once the child gets older. That's why it's so vital for parents to see their children with clear eyes, and if they sense that their kids are developing any of these tendencies, they should take action so that the children don't become stuck in these patterns. The long-term effects of these patterns are not positive for you or your child.

CHAPTER 6: THE LONG ARMS
OF OVERPARENTING

Even when parents are trying their best to kick back, the deluge of appealing electronic tracking and communication devices significantly increases the risk of overparenting at all ages, but especially as our children become adolescents. In fact, new technologies continue to be made available that can provide parents with sophisticated options to improve—and increase—the monitoring of their children. Many child psychologists believe that keeping electronic tabs on our kids can quickly backfire and make things worse. Children often become angry, resentful, and hostile toward parents who don't trust them to stay out of trouble and excessively monitor them. Statistically, kids also are safer on the streets and in schools than ever before, which means that in reality, parents should be breathing a sigh of relief rather than putting their sons and daughters on electronic leashes.[1]

Easier said than done.

The Technology Trap

Parents in the United States are not the only ones who are constantly violating their children's boundaries in their quest to monitor and supervise, if not police, their children. This type of excessive parental behavior is happening all around the world. The *Australian Journal of Guidance and Counseling* reports that schools are struggling with the demands of overly enthusiastic parents. "Experts are saying that the school then becomes responsible for the child having a charmed life," says Queensland University of Technology (Brisbane) PhD researcher Judith Locke. "This is having a huge impact on schools. Not only are schools responsible for teaching students, but they have to manage parents' extreme expectations as well."[2] In essence, parents expect the school to fully monitor and train their children and hold the school accountable if there is any issue with a child.

"In Russia, we have 'The Golden Generation,' children that get everything they point at and then some," says University of Southern Utah student Nikita Ryaschenko about pampering parents in his home country.[3]

According to a 2010 World Economic Forum report on gender equality, sons in Italy are still called *mammomis*, the Italian version of "mama's boy," as they often live at home with their mothers until they turn thirty.[4]

In Hong Kong, private detective Philic Man Hin-nam is seeing a huge increase in the amount of parents hiring her to spy on their children, fearing that their offspring are involved with drugs or trading sexual favors for cash. More often than not, their fears are justified, as Man provides evidence of middle-class, privately educated daughters taking drugs at yacht parties, or thirteen-year-old twin girls from a low-income family engaged in "compensated dating" to buy designer label clothes.

While official figures in Hong Kong suggest that drugs and compensated dating offences have decreased, Man's experience suggests otherwise. She says that her company handled 298 investigations of children in 2011, a 68 percent rise from the 177 cases in 2010. Only twenty-three cases were found to be false alarms.

"Children are more careful now," Man says. "They carry out these activities at home or in a rented room. So they become more 'invisible,' and it's harder for police to catch them." Man also says that her clients are mostly anxious parents who are having difficulty communicating with their children, so they turn to her. She added that in most cases, the children do not know that they were being spied on, and many will never know how they were caught. Man asks her clients not to disclose her evidence to their children and instead refers them to social workers or psychologists on her team.

Social worker Lam Yeung-chu, of the Society of Rehabilitation and Crime Prevention, says that she has reservations about hiring detectives, as it could damage children's relationships with their parents if they ever found out.

"Before they hire detectives, parents should look back and think if there is anything they can do to improve themselves. It is always a bilateral problem," she says.[5] A novel approach might be to try to talk to their children or bring in a third party, such as a counselor.

Similar strife is driving parents to make the same choices in Singapore, where eight out of ten private eye agencies report a rise in parents hiring them to undertake surveillance on their children.

David Ng, director of the private investigation firm DP Quest, says that his company has seen a 20 percent year-on-year increase in requests from parents to check whether their children have gone astray, sometimes even overseas.[6]

"Parents get worried when they see changes in their children's behavior. For example, if they get a tattoo, or start staying out late," he says, explaining the reasons his clients usually cite.

Private eyes usually follow their adolescent subjects for three to five days to glean a pattern. Often, the parents' suspicions are proven right. Their children have been discovered to be involved in illegal activities, such as drugs or gambling. Other times, they are also found at Internet gaming shops late at night without their parents' knowledge.

Video or photographic evidence is then presented to the parents, who decide what to do next. Private investigators say that they start tailing the children as early as when they go to school in the morning.

Joe Koh, from Justice Investigations, says that usually both parents are working and too busy to monitor their children.

For some parents, there is even more reason to track their children when they are studying overseas.

"Parents send us overseas to see how their children are spending their money, and whether they are in relationships," says S. M. Jegan, a private investigator.

Dr. Carol Balhetchet, director of the Singapore Children's Society Youth Service Centre, says, "It's the biggest fear parents have. What is my child up to? But it's very bad for a relationship that's already been contaminated by distrust."[7]

Not to be outdone, private investigators in the United Kingdom are also staying busy tracking teenagers. Belinda Rowlson, of R and L Investigations Services, said there had been "a definite spike in the number of parents wanting their children tailed." She said parents were desperate to find out what their teenagers were getting up to without adult supervision. Often the parents' primary concern is to ensure their teenager avoids violence in nightclubs.

"With the concern about teenagers and alcohol getting out of hand," she said, "we've had parents calling and saying they don't want their children involved in that. They want to make sure their children are safe, and once a parent makes a call to us, word gets around and we get plenty more [cases]."[8]

In Russia, parents often describe themselves as "overprotective" of their children and offer many reasons to explain why. First among these is the general instability of life in a country that saw the powerful state in which most current parents grew up, the USSR, collapse amid social chaos and political strife in the early 1990s.

"Cases of missing children and pedophilia are now covered on TV, and parents' alarm has grown sharply," says Tatiana Gurko, head of family sociology at the official Institute of Sociology in Moscow. "Hyper-protective parents are everywhere. There is a big social discussion going on about whether a law should be passed requiring teenagers to be indoors by a certain hour."[9]

Russian children aren't allowed much freedom. Parents generally accompany their children to school until they're at least twelve, don't let them play on the street or use public transport, and monitor their social lives very closely.

"My daughter Ksenia was twelve when she declared she wanted to go to school by herself and be more independent," Natalya, a single mom who lives in central Moscow told *The Christian Science Monitor*. "Her school was nearby, but she had to cross a busy street to get there. I was worried sick at first, but it worked out. Later I allowed her to go out in the evening with her friends, provided, of course, that I always knew where she was."

Many Russian families also have live-in grandparents, a legacy of Soviet housing shortages, who reinforce the attitude of protectiveness and also provide another layer of supervision for the children.

"Russian parents who consider themselves to be good parents are usually very protective," says Marina Bityanova, head of the independent Tochka Psi psychological center in Moscow. "They have deep-seated fears, which they consider very well-grounded," she adds. "Possibly their surveillance is excessive, but this is the typical Russian reaction. Parents worry that their children may not be able to cope with all the uncertainties and dangers that are out there."[10]

Whether it's in Australia, Moscow, the UK, Hong Kong, or Singapore, when parents go too far with trying to control their children, chances are that it will not end well. The biggest risk is a violation of trust. Naturally, if your child is struggling with a serious issue, such as drug use, sex addiction, or simply running with the wrong crowd, some kind of intervention may be necessary. But for the average teen, it's essential that you take a deep breath, talk to your kid, and try more than anything to build a relationship based on trust. That trust must go both ways, so that you can empower your child to be independent and make good choices while he or she, upon taking that responsibility, can offer you the peace of mind to put your spying equipment back in the closet.

East versus West

In 2011, Yale Law professor Amy Chua created quite a controversy with her *Wall Street Journal* article titled "Why Chinese Mothers Are Superior," citing the benefits of her strict parenting methods, as opposed to the more relaxed Western styles of parenting, which she described as being too lax and an invitation to failure. While some experts praised Chua, many critics considered her philosophy to be harmful to her daughters.

But a subsequent study suggested that it's not merely a question of East versus West, pointing out that family culture is a key to how kids perceive their parents' motivational style.

Chua calls her strict parenting approach "tiger parenting," which prioritizes mastery over effort, while Western parenting focuses more on developing self-esteem and independence. While these approaches reflect cultural differences, they may achieve similar results.[11]

"Parents in both cultures want their children to succeed," said Alyssa Fu, a doctoral student in psychology at Stanford University, at the 2013 meeting of the Society for Personality and Social Psychology.

Fu's research found that Asian American high school kids were more inclined to talk about their mothers' relationships to themselves than were European Americans. Asian Americans tended to mention things such as how their moms helped them with homework or pushed them to succeed, for example. The European Americans were more likely to talk about their mothers as individuals—describing mom's looks or hobbies, for example.

"Asian Americans," Fu said, "see themselves as connected in some way to their mothers. Not even just connected, but their mother is part of who they are."

When it came to how much pressure and support the children felt from their moms, European Americans viewed pressure as a negative. But Asian Americans said pressure and support were not related.

"Asian Americans feel supported by their mothers just as much as the European Americans do, even though they are experiencing more pressure from their mothers," Fu said. "The European American parents provide their children wings so their child can fly away and be free on their own. The Asian American parents are more like the wind that is beneath the wings of their child, because they're always there, supporting the child, letting the child fly and reach success."[12]

The dominant question for parents is this: when pushing your children to succeed academically while being intensely connected to them, can your children still become appropriately independent and eventually function on their own? Or, shall we favor a more laissez faire approach to their academic performance and encourage them to be more independent, in the hopes that they will recognize somewhere along the way that they have to succeed academically and professionally? This is something that each parent and family must decide on their own, taking into account their culture, their surrounding environment, and the personality of their child.

Considering Independent College Counselors

Sending their child to college seems to be the goal for many parents, and selecting the "right" college is the major goal for many of them. In order to make that happen, some families feel that they should hire the services of an independent counselor to increase the likelihood that their children will get into the college of the parents' choice, if not of the children's own choosing. Having experienced the pressures of the college search process on multiple occasions, we understand and sympathize with parents who get stressed out in general with the whole process. But we've also discovered a large group of parents who feel that their situation requires special handling. From all the school counselors we have consulted, it's fair to say that the majority of students do not need the services of what we can only call an exploding cottage industry, better known as the world of tutors. The professional experience and training that most schools provide with their college counseling staff (especially in private schools and charter schools), combined with the support of the administration and faculty, ensure that students receive personalized and accurate guidance, tailored to the individual student throughout the college search process.

The college counselor will write the recommendations that admission officers read, not the independent counselor you hire. Most colleges in this country will not accept recommendations from independent counselors and will not respond to phone calls or emails from an independent counselor about the candidate, a fact that has been underscored in our conversations with college admission officers.

"But what if my daughter gets the added push that an independent counselor can offer, and that ends up making the difference in her getting admitted to the college of her choice?"

Fair enough question, but college admission offices can spot the highly polished, calculated hand of an overcoached application in a heartbeat, and when they do, any hoped-for "advantage" will be lost. The application that might otherwise have been a compelling one if written by the student herself can be relegated very quickly to the "waitlist" or even the "deny" pile. College admission offices see little benefit to students' working with an independent college counselor. In fact, they associate more negatives with that process.

Colleges are looking for a student's authentic voice. They want to know, in students' own words, what they care about, what motivates them, what they think and believe, how they will engage on the campus, and so on. Overly coached and parentally edited applications obliterate the student's voice, leaving the application reader wondering who wrote the essays, who filled out the application, and why this student is particularly interested in the college and would enroll if admitted.

Students will never benefit from the heavy hand of an adult advisor any more than they will from a generic reference by an alumnus who barely knows them. The reason your child gets admitted should be because of his or her efforts and accomplishments. By turning over the process to people who hardly know your child, you risk removing the child's voice, thereby diminishing the success that he or she has achieved through his or her own efforts.

Perhaps a bit of history might be helpful. The profession of independent counseling came into existence as the result of inadequate counseling resources at public high schools. There was a clear need for students and their families to find information about the college process outside of school. But some independent counselors soon learned that there was money to be made in counseling more affluent families who could afford to pay large sums for personal attention. The profession grew even further when it became clear that families were ready to hire on if these independent counselors could tap into the nerve of parental guilt and social pressure.

"If one college counselor is good, two must be better!"

"If I don't pay for an independent counselor, I am not supporting my child."

"Our neighbors have hired a private counselor, so we'd better do it, too."

"Everything I've heard in the news suggests that our child won't get into college without the help of college coaching."

"I don't know anything about the college search process, so we need help!"

For parents with children in private schools, the extra attention and individualized approach, which includes the relationship your child develops with an experienced admission professional, is what some of your tuition is paying for. For those of you with children in public schools, especially large ones, it may be harder to find the same personal attention, but, regardless, the school your child attends is the one with the academic and support personnel dedicated to working with your child throughout the winter and spring of junior year right through to graduation a year later.

School counselors can function in a way that independent counselors cannot. They have full access to school records, teachers, and coaches. They are the source contacted when a college has a question about an applicant. They write the recommendations that most colleges require. Most important, they know the students!

But there are reasons why a family might consider employing an independent counselor. They include a high student-to-counselor ratio, the absence of college counselors and/or college search resources and programs in the school, learning differences (which can vary tremendously from school to school and child to child), Division I and II athletic recruitment, or severe organizational problems with the student or the family.

Whichever direction you choose, based on your child, his or her goals, the school's counseling reputation, and your financial resources, you must try your best to ensure that your child is not caught in the middle of what she is told by the independent counselor and by her school's college counselor. You must also steer clear of allowing an independent counselor to package essays and other responses in a way that makes your child's own voice lost in the final submission. Even worse, do not burden your child with keeping it a secret that he or she is working with an independent counselor. If you do employ an outside counselor, keep the lines of communication open between that person and your school counselor. Having these counselors work in cooperation with each other is in the best interest of your child.

The college admission process is not a contest to be won or a consumer commodity to be bought. As with all things, the college process is an educational journey for your child, one that, with the help of whatever college counselors you work with, will teach your child how to research, make choices, come to know herself, develop lifelong skills that will serve her well, and attain a well-deserved sense of pride and accomplishment when she is offered admission and selects the college of her choice.

However, one caveat worth adding is that you should help your child and the counselor try to find a "hook" that will help differentiate your child from all the other applicants for each spot in the class to which they are applying. It can be athletics, music, theater, or an outside-of-school activity, such as holding down a job to help out with the family income. It really doesn't matter what it is, but it does help for the college to be able to differentiate your child from the others because of your child's individual "hook." The guidance counselor, or whoever writes the recommendations, should know about that as well.

When Parents Can't Let Go

Michael Thompson, coauthor of *Raising Cain: Protecting the Emotional Life of Boys* and author of *Homesick and Happy: How Time Away From Parents Can Help a Child Grow*, discovered during his research that there has been a huge drop in summer-camp attendance over the past generation, and that an increasing number of parents are instead choosing weeklong, skills-based camps. What he found was that those parents who do opt for a longer overnight camp scenario are struggling to say goodbye to their kids. In an earlier generation, the camp would give the children a postcard each week to send home, but in this era some camps provide a constantly updated stream of online photos for these "child-sick" parents.

If parents can't bear to send their kids away to summer camp, and need to keep constant tabs on them when they do, how will they manage when their kids grow up and go to college? Are all the children who left their parents a tearful mess at home now commuting to local community colleges because they feel guilty leaving their parents at home alone? Do children who go away to the college of their parents' choice have their parents rent a house close to their campus so that they can stay in touch more easily, that is, help with their homework and laundry and meals? Hopefully not. If those kids are smart, they'll gently remind their parents to live their own lives and let them live theirs. A compromise would be to put a picture of your child's graduation picture on the refrigerator door or use it as a screensaver on your computer.

But many kids have no such luck, so by the time they leave for college, after having been suffocated, managed, supervised, and maneuvered for their entire childhood, they are out of control as soon as they set foot on campus. They are on their own for the very first time, with no idea what to do or how to monitor or control their behavior. It's akin to watching a child left alone in a candy store with no adult supervision or young men on their first leave from military boot camp. They go wild.

"Every fall," reports a University of Virginia professor, "parents drop off their well-groomed freshmen, and within two or three days many have consumed a dangerous amount of alcohol and placed themselves in harm's way. These kids have been controlled for so long, they just go crazy."

Some parents continue overparenting well into their child's college years by paying for their kids to hire tutors to help them study. Even worse, parents have been known to pay to have their child's papers written for them. In some cases, the college student will hire someone on his or her own, without parental consent. That's what a credit card with unlimited spending and no review of the charges can do. The mistake in either scenario is obvious, but what might the collateral damage be to that child who graduates college with a degree earned entirely by someone else? What kind of moral code does that child have to carry with him for the rest of his life? If any of this sounds at all suspicious, simply check Craigslist on any given day under the "education" heading, and you'll see proof of this illicit industry. The offerings advertise for teachers, writers, and other types of "educators" who are looking to get hired to write papers for undergraduate, graduate, and advanced-level degree students. Is it any wonder that many of these young adults cannot function in a real job, where they are expected to meet someone else's expectations besides those of their parents?

Are some of the current ethical issues that we see in the financial industry a result of this kind of behavior? A student who was recently kicked out of Harvard Law School for falsifying his schoolwork changed his name, went to business school, and was working in finance when he was found to have used illegal insider information to game the system. Was this young man a victim of overparenting?

The Effects of Overparenting on College Graduates

The economic recession of 2008 has had continuing residual effects for many recent college graduates and their families. More and more American college graduates are planning to return to their hometown and move back in with their parents. This is surprising, given the American tradition of kids leaving home as a rite of passage. However, many parents haven't seemed to mind their kids' returning to the family nest. Even though economic circumstances have precipitated much of this, when parents take their kids back into the fold so easily, they are delaying their eventual exit and risking a certain level of arrested development.

Children moving back home can be viewed as a financial safety net for the more than three million so-called "boomerang children" in the United States. But when these short-term stays turn into extended stays, is that a good thing, and is overparenting to blame? Experts disagree on whether the boomerang trend is a good thing, but statistics imply a generational uptick in dependence on parents over the long haul. In 2011, a public opinion poll found that 50 percent of forty-six- to fifty-six-year-old moms financially assisted their adult children, whereas 85 percent of those moms had established financial independence for themselves by twenty-five years of age.[13]

"Whenever possible, it's better for children to live at home for a little longer and become moderately spoiled," says a European-raised mom, now living in Shaker Heights, Ohio. "It is easier to support yourself through school by living with your parents, and, besides, I love getting to make my son's bed again for him." Is this what you want for your twenty-five-year-old?

How does all of this play out for young adults in their twenties and thirties? For parents who have been inclined to overdo it with their kids while raising them, who's to say that they won't continue this behavior with their kids now that they are much older? Parents are still overdoing it with twenty- to thirty-year-old kids. They've been known to go on job interviews with their children, and orchestrate aggressive follow-ups to these meetings. One lawyer responsible for hiring new law school graduates at her firm said that she likes to hire "those who can cope with the everyday demands of our office. Of course, we prefer someone with good grades, but we're always looking for a person who is well-rounded, relative to the quality of their school, someone who can get along with others, think on their feet, and bounce back quickly from any adversity." Obviously, this firm would not be interested in a candidate whose mother accompanies him to the job interview, although that has been known to happen.

Does that "someone" sound like a child who grew up overparented? It's doubtful that many of the children cited here will find lasting success in demanding jobs and/or relationships. At least, it will take them more time to find their way, because overparenting has compromised their development in many key areas. This is not just limited to their career path. It can manifest itself in relationships, where fears of commitment are common, open communication is lacking, and self-esteem is a tenuous affair. None of these conditions, perhaps instigated by an ongoing fear of failure going back to childhood, are conducive to developing healthy relationships that honor commitment and responsibility.

How Overparenting Affects You as a Parent

Children, teachers, and coaches aren't the only ones who pay a price when subjected to overparenting. Parents may lose the most, after all. A mother or father who spends an inordinate amount of time devoted to his or her children may end up with no life of his or her own. Even worse, these parents may experience perpetual angst and guilt from feeling that their children will never survive without them. Or, they may fool themselves into the illusion of being in control (just a false sense of security) of their children's lives, and, thus, of being in control of their own lives. Throw in a rollercoaster of guilt, doubt, and insecurity as their children grow up and leave the nest, and who knows what shape a parent may be in when facing their golden years? Overparenting, while tolerated by children when they are young, takes its biggest toll on parents when it compromises their relationships with their grown children. This is often perpetuated by parents who lavish their kids with expensive cars or even houses that the children could not afford on their own, and then feel resentful when the (adult) child seems unappreciative or angry at them. It is as if they are trying to make one more effort to stay in control and manage everything. And they miss out on some of the best aspects of parenting, as the following story illustrates.

"It is one of the ironies of life," says Paul of Oklahoma City, Oklahoma, "but also very true, I guess, that just when you get what you want, you may not really want it, after all. My son, Jack, was a nutcase as an adolescent, and it seemed like forever until he finished middle school and high school and was ready to go to college. There were times that I felt like one of those guys in prison who was marking the days off on a wall calendar. Then, just before he left, we spent a long weekend together and really enjoyed each other, and I missed him quite badly when he left. All those years I had been there for him, and even though he never showed it, I know now that it meant something to him, and that means everything to me. Sometimes, we don't know the positive effect we have on our children just by hanging around. It's as if we try too hard most of the time because our kids basically function fine without us, as long as we are there."

Choosing a Different Path

More and more parents are resisting the urge to overparent their children and instead are following a path from early on to ensure their child's autonomy. These parents are not rattled by the thought of their child falling from a tree or even breaking a bone in the process because they believe that children need the freedom to explore and learn from their efforts, even if they involve risk.

But as we have stated again and again, along with those risks come subsequent rewards, including newfound creativity, physical exercise, and the sense of empowerment that a child can get from learning something new, all by himself, without the benefit of an adult's helping hands. Children who are given the opportunity to play outdoors unsupervised or to walk or ride a bicycle to school or a friend's house will develop a sense of responsibility, self-esteem, and self-sufficiency. Parents who provide their kids this opening are not negligent, reckless, or uncaring. Most often, they are choosing to create what they consider to be an ideal atmosphere for raising their children. These parents, when they get past the initial anxiety of allowing their children to take the little steps toward independence, also develop a good feeling of having done the right thing as they watch their children flourish. That is very different than manipulating your children to remain dependent on you, which may make you feel very important and central to their lives but will also have the effect of crippling them.

The "Free-Range Kids" movement is a term coined by writer and columnist Lenore Skenazy, whose manifesto on the subject has attracted considerable attention. Skenazy, an op-ed columnist, came into the public eye back in 2008 when she wrote a column about allowing her then-nine-year-old son to ride the New York City subway alone.

"I let him do this because he wanted to take a trip solo, he knew how to read the map, and I had every confidence that he could find his way home," she wrote at the time. "The mere fact that I'd let my son out of my sight made me seem nuts to more than a few people, who wondered why didn't I follow him, or keep checking in with a cell phone, or wait until he was thirty-four and balding before I let him go out on his own."

The backlash continued, which only proved how far the pendulum had swung toward overparenting. A poll on the NBC website asked whether any other viewers would let their kids do what Skenazy had done with hers. Fifty-one percent said no, 20 percent were undecided, and about one-third took Skenazy's side.

Just a generation ago, allowing a child to ride alone on the subway was not considered to be dangerous. Should it be thought of as a threat for that child now, when, according to Congressional Quarterly's 2011 report, New York City has the third-lowest crime rate in America among cities with populations over five hundred thousand? In 2008, the year Skenazy's son rode that train by himself, New York City was ranked 136th in crime overall.[14]

"What my son did is something a whole lot of other city kids do daily," she added, "their mothers are just smart enough not to write about it. I could even add that, believe it or not, I'm a safety fanatic when it comes to helmets and seatbelts."

But children can't wear helmets or seatbelts everywhere they go. Whether you agree with Lenore Skenazy or not, there's no question that we must reconsider the restrictions we choose to place on our children and recognize that at some point they will have to move forward on their own, just as we did once upon a time.

CHAPTER 7: LOOKING FORWARD
AND LETTING GO

If, according to plan, parents guide their children, who, then, guides parents? In the "land of the free and home of the brave" society in which we live and raise our children, the concept of self-help is widely accepted and encouraged. In the parenting world, anyone with a computer can blog his or her best advice, talk-show hosts can peddle their ideas, religious figures from all branches can use their moral authority to intimidate, and licensed professionals can offer tried-and-true solutions based on scientific research that may very well have nothing to do with you or your child. That leaves most of us to our own devices, twisting and turning on our individual quests to do the right thing—if not attain perfection—for our children and ourselves. In reality, though, despite our penchant for trying to appear perpetually confident, we all employ a lot of guesswork, peer consultation (other lost parents), and impulsive decisions along the way. As a result, in order to relieve the parental anxiety of not always knowing what to do with our children, we read books, visit parenting websites, commiserate with our peers, hire consultants, and even see psychiatrists. Once we differentiate between all the contrary opinions and recommendations we have before us and choose a path that we think is right for our situation, we instantly become self-appointed experts, proceeding with great confidence and authority. We tell others of our triumphs but don't usually mention our mistakes. Ironically, this book itself may be a cure for what should be considered a false sense of security.

All joking aside, none of us really knows most of the time what we are doing as parents. Come on. Think about it. We think we do, but we don't. We envision our children as happy, successful little embodiments of ourselves, but is that what we really want for them? Do we even know them? Are we letting them develop into who *they* are, as opposed to who we are trying to mold them to be? Are we giving them the genuine freedom to fumble and fall and find out who they are, while teaching us in the process?

In the pressure-filled world we live in, hounded around the clock by advertising images telling us what we want, what we should look like, what we should do, and what we should aspire to be, do we actually ever step back and take stock of what is most important? If and when we do—other than at times of crisis—do we then authentically share all of that with our children? How do we really know what's best for them? Whether we choose to admit it or not, when it comes to parenting our kids, we are making it up as we go along. So, give yourself a break, and your children, too.

Whose Success Are You Really Seeking?

Many parents will do themselves and their children a great favor by taking a step back and honestly assessing why they are pushing so hard. Whose success are they really after, and at what cost?

In Australia, school psychologists are concerned that overbearing parents are raising children unable to cope with failure and life outside of home, as a new study from Queensland University of Technology in Brisbane shows.[1] A survey of nearly 130 parenting professionals across Australia found that 27 percent had seen "many" instances of overparenting, while almost 65 percent reported having witnessed "some" incidents. Only 8 percent of the psychologists and counselors surveyed reported no incidents of overparenting.

But because overparenting is a spectrum phenomenon, even reasonable, relatively well-adjusted parents who have been doing a good job of raising their children may slide into the yellow or red zone during a time of crisis, at least for a short period of time until the problem is resolved, which in and of itself is not a bad thing.

PhD researcher Judith Locke, a clinical psychologist affiliated with Queensland University of Technology in Australia, says, "Parents are typically doing the best job they can do, and this type of parenting is done with the best of intentions and out of love. However, more effort doesn't necessarily produce a better child. There may be a point at which effort can become harmful. Parenting professionals are concerned that overparenting reduces a child's resilience and life skills because they've never had to face any difficulties. It could also create a sense of entitlement in children. If they have someone constantly making their life perfect, they expect everybody to make their life perfect for them."[2]

While overparenting can be a problem on many levels, it also has a good side: the children of these moms and dads are lucky enough to have parents who are diligent, attentive, and caring, even if they might go overboard. Finding a middle ground between too much and too little is not as easy as it may sound, but a little objectivity can go a long way.

Many parents start out with overanxious tendencies, but as they gather experience and confidence they tend to relax and settle in to the wonderful job of parenting. This is particularly the case after the first or second child.

A good place to begin is accepting—and loving— your kids for who they are, not what you wish they would be. Whether you have grand ideas about your child excelling in the classroom, on stage, or in a stadium full of fans as an athlete, you might want to reconsider *why* these things are so important to you. Cooling your expectations and just enjoying your kid for who he or she is and what he or she likes will relieve you and your child of a lot of needless anxiety. That will put you on a solid track toward good parenting. And allowing your child to experience frustration, confusion, or plain old failure is not a bad thing at all. Whatever shortcomings your child experiences do not constitute a negative reflection on you. In fact, you will do your kid a favor when you stay out of the way and let him or her negotiate his or her own way—in school, around the neighborhood, and in life in general. Just think of it as a learning experience for both of you.

Next time your son gets a disappointing grade, will you be able to keep yourself from emailing his teacher? If your daughter loses her starting position on her school soccer team, will you keep your mouth shut with other parents and her coach? As Victoria Clayton, coauthor of *Fearless Pregnancy: Wisdom and Reassurance from a Doctor, a Midwife and a Mom*,[3] says on nbcnews.com, "Remember, the world will continue to exist even if your child fails his French test."[4] That's right. One test does not define a résumé, someone's character, or your kid's potential. Give yourself a break, and don't let every up and down define your day.

Through the Looking Glass:
A Personal Note from George S. Glass, MD

Since fathering my first child more than forty years ago, adding two stepchildren some years later, and then two more twenty-five years ago, I've experienced firsthand the bumpy and wondrous road of parenting. When you add in the thousands of patients I've treated in my psychiatric practice who are struggling with an assortment of parenting issues, you could say that I've learned quite a bit, often as much (or more) from my own mistakes (as my children like to point out) as from those I've seen in others.

Here's the upshot of it all: we all want to see our children succeed—at every level. Whether it's your five-year-old playing a tree in a school play, your seven-year-old entering a spelling bee, or your ten-year-old pitching in a baseball game, you want to see your child doing well. Sometimes, in fact, parents may go so far as to pressure their children to excel in an activity that's supposed to be breezy and fun.

Sound familiar? Have you ever rehearsed your child, over and over, to make sure that he or she played that tree just right? Do you know someone who hired a tutor to coach their second-grader for a school spelling bee?

Unfortunately, many parents need to take a step back and honestly assess why they are pushing their kids so hard. Whose success are they really after, and at what cost, literally and figuratively? Honestly, are you wishing for your child's success or yours? If your son forgets his lines, misspells a word, or throws a wild pitch, how does that make you feel? Whose self-esteem is really at stake? Will the other parents look at you as a "bad parent" because of that? In my professional experience, children who have an extracurricular activity they like and can begin to excel in feel better about themselves, which in turn helps build their self-esteem. They feel special because of their efforts, not simply because they feel entitled to be successful or because you hired a coach or tutor to get them to that point. If they enjoy it and continue, they feel better, and that increases their sense of self-worth. That helps them do better in school as well as in other areas of their life, and they are less likely to get into drugs. They don't have to be a star, but they need to know that you support and encourage them in whatever they have chosen to do. If you repeatedly don't show up, and you don't have a clear reason that you explain, the message you give your children is that you don't really care about them or what they do, that whatever you are doing is more important to you than they are.

As a parent, it is your job to be there, ready, willing, and able, when your child wants to talk and be listened to *without* being judged or pressured to change. It is best to suggest ideas only when your child seems to be in a receptive mood. If you just jump in, intending to fix things, it will invariably backfire. Your desire to rectify a challenging situation may be admirable, but your child needs to learn how to deal with life on his or her own terms. Being there to listen is important—all by itself. You don't always have to try to teach your child a new lesson with every discussion you have with him or her. While you may think that your child should already know this or that, he or she may not be ready to learn, at least not from you. That realization can be intense for a parent and a tough pill to swallow, but trust your child more often than not to figure things out on his or her own. And know that your presence is worth something, without your becoming the "fixer." Besides, if you are available, if not there all the time, your children will be more comfortable coming to you, if and when they do have issues. At those times, they will also listen and be more likely to take your advice.

No simple set of rules or techniques will work in every situation, even if they've often worked before. Circumstances change, communication varies, and children respond differently as they grow older. This means that all of us will continue making mistakes. Some may even horrify us when we think back and remember doing things that we wish in retrospect we had never done, or can't believe we actually did.

This can be avoided in large part by not trying so hard. Your kids generally know that you love them and care about them. It is not necessary to thrust yourself into the middle of everything they do, or try to be a super-parent in an effort to get them to like you or make up for what you perceive to be inadequacies in your overall parenting or in their lives. It is enough to be present and involved when appropriate.

The secret is giving your time, commitment, and consistency.

A Prescription for Healthy Parenting

Once your first child is born, you are faced with one choice after another, and it's not easy to know whether you are making the right ones, let alone the best ones for your kid, who you are still getting to know—one day at a time. But there are some basics to follow, and these prescriptive guidelines will help you make good choices.

1. When it comes to your kids, spend time before money.
2. Listen to their wishes before sharing yours. Support *their* interests, not yours. If they end up not liking something, let *them* decide.
3. Let your kids fail, beginning with the first time they fall down on the playground. They need to learn early on that life is full of bumps and bruises, and that they have the wherewithal to overcome them. *Remember: Small kids = Small problems. Big kids = Big problems.*
4. Work with your children on how they can learn from their mistakes. Mistakes can often be opportunities, which can lead to positive problem-solving skills.
5. Let them take pride in *their* creations, even if you think they should be "better." It's *their* science fair. You had yours.

6. For the most part, let your kids pick their own friends. This develops their emotional intelligence and social awareness.

7. Encourage your child to deal directly with his or her own teacher. Negotiation is an essential—and ongoing—skill for your child to develop.

8. Do not overschedule your children. They need time to reflect, because, even if you don't realize it, life is happening quite quickly for them, too.

9. Embrace free time with nothing specific to do. This is when you can find each other as parent and child, with nothing on anyone's agenda!

10. Let go.

A Cautionary Tale from the Tabatsky Files

What if your kid is like me, and when he's four, he thinks he's Superman and tries to fly down a flight of stairs and breaks his collarbone (which still hurts when it rains)? What should my parents have done to prevent that? What could they have done to turn off my imagination? Chain me to the radiator in my room? I suppose I blame them for letting me watch *Superman* on TV in the first place. I can also blame my mother for safety-pinning a dishtowel to my back as a cape. Being an innocent child, both indulgences obviously made me susceptible to seeking adventure and vulnerable to the foibles of such a pursuit. Children should never be subjected to that, right? Gosh, what was wrong with my parents? Had they no sense of what the big, bad world was all about, especially the one in our very own home? George? Are you there? I think I need help. I think I should revisit my childhood and find out what was really going on between my parents and me. Or maybe it was my sister; maybe she pushed me down the stairs just to see what would happen. Well, I'll tell you what happened. I learned what risk is all about, how it involves pain and pleasure and most of all—living! I should thank my parents. I don't need therapy. I just need to remember the value in that whole incident and move on with my life. I may even buy a Superman T-shirt and go skydiving with my sister.

The Trickle-Down Effects of Stay-at-Home Dads

If fathers took paternity leave more often, which is slowly becoming a growing phenomenon in the United States, overparenting would decrease. We're just suggesting this, because logic would have it that when men use the paternity leave they have coming to them, three things can happen:

1. Fathers become more engaged and active at home with childcare, housekeeping, and general maintenance. They might even cultivate a hobby that doesn't include sports or finances.

2. Mothers, then, have a chance to become more invested in their careers and with whatever else they had no time to do before Dad got involved around the house and with the kids. They don't necessarily get a life, but they enhance the one they already have.

3. Children get the best of both parents, because each of them is more relaxed, less anxious, and genuinely appreciative of the new family dynamics.

Everybody wins.

Not everyone can reap the benefits of time away from work when a new baby is born, however. The federal Family and Medical Leave Act has been around a long time, guaranteeing up to twelve weeks of *unpaid* leave to new mothers and fathers who work in large and medium-sized workplaces. In 2002, California became the first state to guarantee six weeks of *paid* leave for moms and dads, and Rhode

Island and New Jersey have subsequently adopted their own versions of the law. Some of the tech giants in Silicon Valley have become even more generous. Google and Yahoo offer men seven and eight weeks, respectively, while Reddit and Facebook have pushed the number to seventeen.[5]

When men take time to be home with their child, leaving women more time to be at work, it's better for the economy, because with more women maintaining their vital positions in the workforce, companies function more effectively and women can continue to build their roles in the corporate structure.

University of Oregon sociologist Scott Coltrane notes that when men share "routine repetitive chores," women feel that they are being treated fairly and are less likely to become depressed.[6]

When that occurs, when mothers and fathers are less stressed, are less anxious, and feel less guilt for being away so much, common sense says that they will be better parents. The main reason for that would be that they would not be putting undue pressure on themselves or their children. As a result, they would also be less prone to overcompensating, overdoing their involvement, and overparenting. In general, they would have a life outside of just the house and the kids.

What Children Really Want Their Parents to Do with Them

If you ask a typical elementary school class what they want most from their parents, you may be surprised by their answers.[7] Even in the material world in which we live, most of the kids did not choose iPads and games and the latest popular shoes. Instead, they showed a decided preference for parents being there, paying attention, and helping when they were asked. Those things made them feel safe, secure, and loved, the unofficial "Big Three" of basic universal human needs. It would probably be a very safe bet that this has not changed at all since something like forever.

Sure, kids like presents. We all do. But those usually appear on birthdays and special holidays, and should suffice. Kids need things from unreachable shelves, too; they enjoy their favorite foods, and they want to be driven places; but at the end of the day—literally— what they want most is a parent who is able and willing to just hang out.

So, why are so many moms and dads convinced that they are not being good parents unless they are racing around, bouncing their kids from one activity to another, fearful that their children might be missing something crucial in their life development?

Little kids love it most when their parents cuddle up with them to read and tell them stories. It gets even better when the lights go out and you can share dreams and fears together. That intimate time can never compete with a TV show. And if you have more than one child, try to find time for that one-on-one time with each one of your kids.

As they get older, dinner table conversations can become very grounding, especially if they're not limited to school talk. That's also a time when parents can extend the leash and let kids play outside without constant supervision. It's not only exciting for your kids. It's liberating!

At almost any age (aside from those terrible twos), kids actually want limits, and when you establish rules and enforce them fairly, you are showing real love and devotion. When kids don't have rules and limits, they often make up their own, which can be much stricter than anything their parents would devise.

Up until the middle school years, most kids like it when their parents hide little notes in their backpacks and lunchboxes. You may want to stop doing that when they reach their teen years, as that kind of love can quickly become too much. But care packages are much appreciated all over again once your kid goes off to college.

Do we sometimes forget that our children are pretty smart, and that it happens totally without us, or even in spite of us? It behooves us to tap into their brains and see what we can learn from them, if we let them talk and are willing to listen when they do.

The old adage that children keep you young is not just because you are chasing after them, but because they bring you fresh ideas, new ways to look at things, and alternative methods for approaching situations that you never considered; as a result of getting so set in your ways, you sometimes forget that life can be approached differently.

The Parenting Paradox

Dr. Bob Moorehead, a graduate of the California School of Theology and the former pastor of Overlake Christian Church in Redmond, Washington, preached about how we have progressed as a society, with bigger buildings, faster planes and an endless amount of conveniences, but as people, we may be enjoying life less instead of more.

Parents today get easily caught up in a whirlwind of activities aimed at exposing their children to the world, supposedly making them ready to succeed. But at what cost? When we equip our children to make a living, are we also giving them the tools to live a life of quality and love? We can send people to the moon, but can we take care of our spiritual needs right here at home? As our lives speed up, what lessons are we teaching our children about slowing down to appreciate what's right in front of them? For example, fast food is easy and convenient, but there's nothing like a slow-cooked dish, made with care and love, right at home. And, caught up in our very important and busy lives, we all can opt out and send an email or a text to a friend or family member, forfeiting what could be an intimate moment on the telephone or, even better, an actual visit in person.

Most of all, with life seeming to race by at faster and faster speeds, parents are challenged to let go and allow their children to find things out for themselves, with a certain amount of failure to be expected in the mix of growing up.

So how do we deal with the paradox of parenting?

D. H. Lawrence offered some sage advice back in 1918: "How to begin to educate a child. First rule: leave him alone. Second rule: leave him alone. Third rule: leave him alone. That is the whole beginning."[8]

And, in the words of Luke Skywalker, "May the force be with you."

Parental Aptitude Test Answers

(from pages 78–80)

1. Successful parenting means:
    C. Your children enjoy growing up and feel good about themselves.
2. Children should be seen, heard, or tested.
    D. All of the above (but "tested" we recommend only on an occasional basis.)
3. If your child breastfeeds, it means that he will:
    D. Never go hungry.
4. Love means never having to say:
    D. None of the above.
5. If your child fails a math test in third grade, it means:
    D. None of the above.
6. When your son's soccer coach doesn't start your son, you react by:
    D. Enjoying the game.
7. When your daughter wins an award for the sixth-grade science fair, you:
    A. Tell her that you're proud of her.
8. Your child is not sure whether he wants to go to college. This make you feel:
    D. Curious. Why does he feel that way?
9. If your son is being bullied by his seventh-grade classmates, what do you do?
    C. Ask your son what's happening.
10. When your five-year-old falls off a sliding board and breaks his arm, you choose to:
    D. None of the above.

ACKNOWLEDGMENTS

We would like to thank Francine Edelman, our agent, who encouraged us to take on this project. Thanks to James Racheff for his diligent research and administrative help.

Thanks to all of the teachers, administrative staff and school leaders whose insights and stories played a significant role in shaping this book. We are deeply indebted to those individuals around the country who have spent their life primarily educating children and adolescents, and whose work clearly involved engaging with and imparting knowledge to many of the parents of their disciples.

We would especially like to thank a number of folks in the Houston, Texas, area whose contributions were invaluable: Dr. Lue Bishop, Dean and Head of the Upper School and Ms. Lyn Slaughter, Director of College Counseling at the Emery Weiner School, Elaine Eichelberger, Dean of Students, Deborah Whalen, Principal, Debbie Skelly, Director of Guidance, and Kim Scoville, Academic Dean of the St. Agnes School, and Ms. Helen Vietor, the director of the Pooh Corner Preschool for over sixty-one years.

We'd like to extend a special acknowledgment to the educational professionals, developmental specialists and parents who spoke to us anonymously and informally. Their viewpoints and perspectives have helped enormously to shape this book. They include Sam, Alicia and Danny, Mo and Bette, Dan and Angel, Joan, Mimi and Cindy,

Diane, Jane, Samantha, Sylvia, Chris, Ingrid, Norris, Simon and Dee, Melody and Bill, Benjy, Cynthia, Morgan, Ben, Tabitha, Ray, Brian, Claudia, Kevin, Meg, Robert, Vicky, Jessica and Crystal, Ritu, Sanji, Priti, Allison, Suzi, Karen, Molly, Mrs. Brando, Trent, Kim, Igarashi, Jamie, Larry, Luanne, Lauren and Crissy and Paul.

George S. Glass
I am indebted to my wife, Donna Glass, who allowed me to take time and energy away from her and our family life to work on this while also doing my day job as a psychiatrist. I also want to thank my five children and four grandchildren, who are still talking to me although from early on they tried to educate me about my own failings as a helicopter parent. I would go on to single out our daughter, Rebecca Robinson, and her high school friend, Grace Ebaugh, who were willing to share with us their common and individual experiences as children and parents.

Last but not least, I had ongoing input and support from a number of my mental health colleagues including Joan Anderson, PhD., Jean Guez, PhD., Morton Katz, PhD., and Milton Altschuler, MD.

David Tabatsky
I am grateful to George Glass for his camaraderie, good spirit and encouragement, and to Donna for her consistently gracious hospitality.

Thanks to Dr. Mark Banschick, my coauthor on *The Intelligent Divorce*, for his knowledge and continuing support. Thanks to the parents and educators of The Calhoun School for their assistance.

Finally, thank you to my children, Max and Stella, who have personally shown me—sometimes in great detail—what overparenting can be.

ABOUT THE AUTHORS

George S. Glass, MD

George S. Glass is a father and grandfather. He has served as a medical doctor and psychiatrist for more than thirty years. He received a bachelor's degree in psychology from Swarthmore College, earned a medical degree from Northwestern University Medical School in Chicago, and did his psychiatric residency at the Yale University Medical School. He is a board-certified psychiatrist and addictionologist.

Dr. Glass's post-residency training included intensive studies of the treatment of alcoholism and substance abuse, which led to clinical experience in the treatment of adult, adolescent, and geriatric individuals with psychiatric and substance abuse problems, including alcohol- and drug-related issues, depression, and issues resulting from physical, psychological, and stress-related traumas, including divorce.

Since 1986, he has been helping families, attorneys, and courts deal with the psychological consequences of divorce. Dr. Glass has traveled throughout Texas as a forensic expert in family court cases, as well as conducting group presentations and divorce workshops, and treating patients involved in family disruptions.

Dr. Glass has administered, owned, and directed inpatient hospital treatment programs, day hospital programs, a community mental health center, and a residential treatment center, beginning in 1972 when he set up the US Navy's first alcohol treatment program at the Bethesda Naval Hospital, and he has since served as chairman of departments of psychiatry at several Houston hospitals.

Dr. Glass's academic credits include appointments as a clinical associate professor of psychiatry at the Baylor College of Medicine and the University of Texas Medical School and School of Public Health and the Cornell Weill School of Medicine.

Dr. Glass has developed, managed, and conducted independent medical evaluations for the FAA, the Airline Pilot's Association, Harris County Medical Society, the Texas State Bar, multiple Fortune 500 companies and their unions, as well as federal, state, and local courts and attorneys who work with them.

Please visit www.GeorgeSGlassMDPA.com for more information.

David Tabatsky

David Tabatsky is a single father of two children, one halfway through college and the other about to leave home very soon. When he is not wandering about aimlessly, pining for his son and daughter, he is a writer, editor, teacher, director, and performing artist. He received his bachelor's degree in communications and a master's degree in theater education, both from Adelphi University.

Tabatsky is the author of *Write for Life: Communicating Your Way Through Cancer* (2013) and coauthor of *The Cancer Book: 101 Stories of Courage, Support and Love* and editor of Elizabeth Bayer's *It's Just a Word*, both published by Chicken Soup for the Soul Publishing in 2009. He is the coauthor, with Bruce Kluger, of *Dear President Obama: Letters of Hope from Children Across America*, also published in 2009. Tabatsky wrote *The Boy Behind the Door: How Salomon Kool Escaped the Nazis* (2009). With Dr. Mark Banschick, Tabatsky coauthored

The Intelligent Divorce—Books One and Two (2009 and 2010) and *The Wright Choice: Your Family's Guide to Healthy Eating, Modern Fitness and Saving Money* (2011), with Dr. Randy Wright. Tabatsky was the consulting editor for Marlo Thomas and her *New York Times* bestseller *The Right Words at the Right Time, Volume 2: Your Turn* (2006). He has published two editions of *What's Cool Berlin*, a comic travel guide to Germany's capital, and has written for *The Forward*, *Parenting*, and *Sesame Street Parent*, among other publications.

Tabatsky has worked professionally in theater and circus as an actor, clown, and juggler, at Lincoln Center, Radio City Music Hall, and the Beacon Theatre, and throughout the United States and Europe, most notably at the Chamäleon in Berlin, New End Theatre in London, Folies Pigalle in Paris, and the Edinburgh Fringe Festival, where *The Stage* wrote, "He is a supremely skillful performer and a fine actor, reaching levels no other comics have matched at this Fringe." Tabatsky also directed Kinderzirkus Taborka at the renowned Tempodrom in Berlin.

Tabatsky has taught for the American School of London, die Etage in Berlin, the Big Apple Circus School, the United Nations International School, and the Cathedral of St. John the Divine. He served on the theater faculty at Adelphi University and the Cooper Union and as a teaching artist for the Henry Street Settlement, with a focus on special education. He teaches circus arts at Sunrise Day Camp, America's only dedicated day camp for children with cancer and their siblings.

Please visit www.tabatsky.com and www.writeforlife.info for more information.

NOTES

Introduction
[1] Jennifer Finney Boylan, "The Risk Pool," in Op-Ed, *The New York Times*, August 27, 2013

Chapter 1
[1] Madaline Levine, "Raising Successful Children," Sunday Review; The Opinion Pages, *The New York Times*, August 5, 2012.

Chapter 2
[1] Susan Guibert, "Research shows child rearing practices of distant ancestors foster morality and compassion in kids," University of Notre Dame, *Notre Dame News*, September 17, 2010, http://www.news.nd.edu/news/168.

[2] Robert Francis Harper, ed. "Some Babylonian Laws" in *Assyrian and Bablonian Literature*, William Muss-Arnolt, tran. (New York, D. Appleton and Company, 1904).

[3] J. B. Watson, *Psychological Care of Infant and Child* (New York: W. W. Norton & Co., 1928).

[4] A. S. Neil, *Summerhill: A Radical Approach to Child Rearing* (New York: Hart Publishing Company, 1960).

[5] *Summerhill: A Radical Approach.*

[6] Diana Baumrind, "Effects of Authoritarian Parental Control on Child Behavior," *Child Development*, No. 37 (1968), 887-907.

7   Suzanne M. Bianchi, John P. Robinson, Melissa A. Milke, *The Changing Rhythms of American Family Life* (New York, Russell Sage Foundation, 2006).

8   Diana Baumrind, "Effects of Authoritarian Parental Control on Child Behavior," *Child Development,* 37 (1968), 887-907.

9   "N.Y. school bans balls at recess, cracks down on tag games over safety fears," Ryan Jaslow, *CBS News* (New York: WCBS, October 8, 2013).

10 Nancy Gibbs, "The Growing Backlash Against Overparenting," *Time* (November 30, 2009), http://www.time.com/time/nation/article/0,8599,1940395,00.html.

Chapter 3

1   Cristen Conger, "5 Signs of Overparenting," howstuffworks.com, (June 21, 2014) http://www.howstuffworks.com/5-signs-of-over-parenting2.htm.

2   Magid, Larry, "Is Taser Guilty of Over-Parenting?" *CBS News,* January 13, 2010. (April 17, 2012) http://www.cbsnews.com/2100-500163_162-6091550.htm.

3   Brett Singer, "Apps for Paranoid Parents," Parents.com. January 20, 2012 (April 17, 2012) http://shine.yahoo.com/parenting/apps-paranoid-parents-145600007.html.

4   Nick Gillespie, "Stop Panicking About Bullies," *Wall Street Journal,* (April 2, 2012).

5   Ata Johnson, "The Professional Kid—Too Big To Fail?", *TheRockmomblog,* therockmom.com (January 16, 2013), http://www.therockmom.com/2013/01.

6   Carl Honoré, *Under Pressure: Rescuing Our Children from the Culture of Hyper-Parenting* (New York: HarperOne Reprint Edition, 2009).

7   Dylan Matthews, "The key to evaluating teachers: Ask kids what they think," *wonkblog,* washingtonpost.com (February 23, 2013), http://

www.washingtonpost.com/blogs/wonkblog/wp/2013/02/23/
the-key-to-evaluating-teachers-ask-kids-what-they-think.

8   George Carlin, *You Are All Diseased*, Atlantic Records, released
    May 18, 1999.

9   "Drawbacks of Overprotective Parents," IndiaParenting.com,
    http://www.indiaparenting.com/raising-children/128_913/draw-
    backs-of-overprotective-parents.html.

10 Ata Johnson, "The Professional Kid—Too Big To Fail?",
    TheRockmomblog, therockmom.com (January 16, 2013) http://
    www.therockmom.com/2013/01.

11 P. Solomon Banda, "Aggressive Parents Force Colorado Egg Hunt
    Cancellation," Huffingtonpost.com (March 26, 2012), http://www.
    huffingtonpost.com/2012/03/26/colorado-egg-hunt_n_1379226.
    html.

12 "Get families talking about separating," nctmums.com, http://
    www.netmums.com/home/netmums-campaigns/get-families-
    talking-about-separating.

13 Stephen T. Asma, *Against Fairness*, (Chicago, IL: University of
    Chicago Press, 2012).

Chapter 4

1   "Survey of high school athletes: 2006," Josephson Institute Center
    for Sports Ethics," (2006), http://josephsoninstitute.org/sports/
    programs/survey.

2   Michael De Groot, "Gotta have: Are smartphones a need or
    just a want?" *Deseret News*, National Edition, October 16, 2013,
    http://national.deseretnews.com/article/472/Gotta-have-Are-
    smartphones-a-need-or-just-a-want.html.

3   Louis C.K., September 23, 2013, "Conan", TBS.

4   Howard P. Chudacoff, *Children at Play: An American History*,
    (New York and London: New York University Press, 2007).

5   Peter Gray, "The Play Deficit: Children today are cossetted and pressured in equal measure. Without the freedom to play they will never grow up," *Aeon Magazine* (September 18, 2013), http://aeon.co/magazine/being-human/children-today-are-suffering-a-severe-deficit-of-play.

6   Lizette Alvarez, "Felony Counts for 2 in Suicide of Bullied 12-Year-Old," *The New York Times*, October 16, 2013.

7   "Poor parenting – including overprotection – increases bullying risk, study of 200,000 children shows", *Warwick News and Events* http://www2.warwick.ac.uk/newsandevents/pressreleases/poor_parenting_150.

8   Catherine Saint Louis, "Effects of Bullying Last into Adulthood, Study Finds", *The New York Times*, February 21, 2013, page A15.

9   William E. Copeland, Dieter Wolke, Adrian Angold, E. Jane Costello, "Adult Psychiatric Outcomes of Bullying and Being Bullied by Peers in Childhood and Adolescence", *JAMA Psychiatry*, http://archpsyc.jamanetwork.com/article.aspx?articleid=1654916.

10 Amanda Ripley, "The Case Against High School Sports", *The Atlantic*, October 2013.

11 Amanda Ripley, "The Case Against High School Sports", *The Atlantic*, October 2013.

12 "The Case Against High School Sports."

13 *Honey Grove Preservation League*, http://www.honeygrovepreservation.org/wall-school.html.

14 "The Case Against High School Sports."

15 Diana Nyad, "Views of Sport; How Illiteracy Makes Athletes Run," *The New York Times*, May 28, 1989.

16 "Is Your Child Ready for Sports? (Care of the Young Athlete)," *American Academy of Pediatrics, Patient Education Online*, http://patiented.aap.org/content2.aspx?aid=7354.

17 Amanda Williams, "Pressure on Kids in Sports," *Live Strong Foundation*, Livestrong.com (updated October 21, 2013), http://www.livestrong.com/article/78818-pressure-kids-sports.

Chapter 5

1 Doan Bui, "From China to France to America, a Backlash Against Overparenting," *Worldcrunch.com* (January 24, 2013), http://www.worldcrunch.com/culture-society/from-china-to-france-to-america-a-backlash-against-overprotective-parents/parenting-children-overparenting-helicopter-chua-druckerman/c3s10713.

2 Jakob Asplund, "Overprotective parenting a growing worldwide problem," *Hard News Café*, Logan Library (December 12, 2010), http://www.hardnewscafe.usu.edu/?p=3509.

3 "Overprotective parenting a growing worldwide problem."

4 Katherine Ozment, "Welcome to the Age of Overparenting", *Boston Magazine,* December 2011.

5 Steve Baskin, "The Gift of Failure," *Psychology Today* (December 31, 2011).

6 Nathaniel Branden, *The Psychology of Self-Esteem: A Revolutionary Approach to Self-Understanding that Launched a New Era in Modern Psychology,* (New York: Tarcher, 1969).

7 "5 Signs of Overparenting."

8 Lori Gottlieb, "How to Land Your Kid in Therapy", *The Atlantic*, July 2011.

9 Peter Gray, "The Decline of Play and the Rise of Psychopathology in Children and Adolescents," *American Journal of Play*, Volume 3, Number 4, Spring (2011).

10 Sandra L. Hofferth, "Changes in American children's time – 1997 to 2003," *PubMed Central (PMC)*, *Electronic International Journal*

of Time Use Research. Author manuscript; available in *PMC*,
September 15, 2010, published in final edited form as: *Electronic
International Journal of Time Use Research.* January 1, 2009; 6(1):
26–47.

11 Jamie Hale, "Interview with Margarita Tartakovsky," *World of
Psychology Blog,* PsychCentral.com (February 8, 2012), http://
psychcentral.com/blog/archives/2012/02/08/interview-with-
margarita-tartakovsky.

12 Bruno Bettelheim, "The Importance of Play," *The Atlantic Monthly,*
March 1987.

13 "Welcome to the Age of Overparenting."

14 "Anxiety Disorders in Children," ADAA.org, http://www.adaa.
org/sites/default/files/Anxiety%20Disorders%20in%20Children.
pdf.

15 Vanessa van Petten, "10 Qualities of Teacup Parenting: Is Your Kid
Too Fragile?", *Radical Parenting* (June 19, 2008), http://www.radi-
calparenting.com/2008/06/19/10-qualities-of-teacup-parenting-
is-your-kid-too-fragile.

16 Wendy Mogel, "The Dark Side of Parental Devotion: How Camp
Can Let the Sun Shine," *Camping Magazine* (2006: January/
February).

17 "10 Qualities of Teacup Parenting."

18 "The Dark Side of Parental Devotion."

19 "The Dark Side of Parental Devotion."

Chapter 6

1 Nick Gillespie, "Stop Panicking About Bullies," *Wall Street Journal,*
April 02, 2012 (April 17, 2012), http://online.wsj.com/article/SB1
0001424052702303404704577311664105746848.html.

2 "Overprotective parenting a growing worldwide problem."

3   "Overprotective parenting a growing worldwide problem."

4   "Overprotective parenting a growing worldwide problem."

5   Simon Cheung, "Wary parents hire private eye for kids", *South China Morning Post*, June 11, 2012.

6   "Wary parents hire private eye for kids."

7   Jalelah Abu Bakar, "More parents hiring private eyes to check on their kids," *The Straits Times*, October 16, 2013.

8   Sean Thompson, "Sleuths track rowdy teens – parents keep an eye on schoolies," *The Daily Telegraph*, page 15, November 30, 2013.

9   Fred Weir, "Russian parents make no apologies for being 'hyper-protective'," *The Christian Science Monitor*, May 22, 2013.

10   "Russian parents make no apologies for being 'hyperprotective'."

11   Stephanie Pappas, "'Tiger Mom' & Her Critics Both Right, Study Finds," *Livescience*, January 22, 2013, http://www.livescience.com/26465-tiger-parenting-cultural-style.html.

12   "'Tiger Mom' & Her Critics Both Right, Study Finds."

13   Barabra Liston, "Many U.S. baby boomer mums support grown kids – poll," *Reuters, Edition UK*, April 15, 2011, http://uk.reuters.com/article/2011/04/15/oukoc uk-boomers-mothers-idUKTRE73E4U120110415.

14   Lenore Skenazy, "Why I'm Raising Free-Range Kids," the Blog, *Huffington Post* (New York), U.S. Edition, June 24, 2009.

Chapter 7

1   "Overparenting trend worries psychologists," Queensland University of Technology, *Medical Xpress* (January 15, 2013), http://medicalxpress.com/news/2013-01-overparenting-trend-psychologists.html.

2   Pilar Onatra, "Over parenting: When caring too much becomes harmful," *BC Council for Families,* February 14, 2014

3 Victoria Clayton, Stuart Fischbein, Joyce Weckl, *"Fearless Pregnancy: Wisdom and Reassurance from a Doctor, a Midwife and a Mom,"* (Beverly, MA: Fair Winds Press, 2004).

4 Victoria Clayton, "Overparenting: When good intentions go too far, kids can suffer", *nbcnews.com* (December 7, 2004), http://www.nbcnews.com/id/6620793/ns/health-childrens_health/t/overparenting/#.U6n8Tj3YImk.

5 Liza Mundy, "Daddy Track: The Case for Paternity Leave," *The Atlantic*, January/February 2014.

6 "Daddy Track: The Case for Paternity Leave."

7 Erin Kurt, "The Top 10 Things Children Really Want Their Parents To Do With Them," *Lifehack*, lifehack.org, http://www.lifehack.org/articles/lifestyle/the-top-10-things-children-really-want-their-parents-to-do-with-them.html.

8 D. H. Lawrence, "Education of the People" essay, *Times Educational Supplement* (circa 1918).